Understanding the Grief and Loss Experiences of Carers

This book draws on recent research and cutting-edge ideas about bereavement and carers' experiences across the life course to explore carers' experience of loss and discuss their specific needs prior and or following the death of those they care for.

Whether care provided is related to a long term or life limiting condition, many carers experience a multitude of losses including indefinite loss characterised by the loss of a taken-for-granted future, and an inability to plan for the future. Carers may also experience anticipatory grief as multiple losses such as companionship, personal freedom, and control manifest. While many carers are dedicated and committed to their role, they are subject to burnout and disenfranchised grief. When the role of caregiver ends as a result of the death of those cared for, this can represent a major change and a period of significant adjustment for carers leading to a range of emotions experienced.

This book presents and discusses research findings, practitioner perspectives, and a wealth of personal accounts to illuminate this vital but neglected area and extend our understanding of loss for carers across the life course. This interdisciplinary and interprofessional volume brings together authors from a wide range of backgrounds, including carers themselves. It is an important contribution to the burgeoning literature around the role and experiences of carers and will interest academics, students and practitioners in health and social care, counselling, and psychology with an interest in loss and bereavement.

Kerry Jones is a Senior Lecturer at The Open University, UK, where her research and teaching focus on death, dying, grief, bereavement and end-of-life care. As Co-Lead of the Open University Carers Research Group, she has published and presented her research on care homes and care-giving staff during the pandemic, stillbirth neonatal death, parental bereavement, brain injury, dementia and suicide. Kerry was an academic consultant for *A Time to Live* on BBC 2.

Joanna Horne is a Senior Lecturer in Psychology and Counselling at The Open University, UK. She conducts research within the areas of physical activity and carer wellbeing, and support needs of young carers. Jo is a member of the Open University Carers Research Group.

Routledge Key Themes in Health and Society

Available titles include:

Partiality and Justice in Nursing Care
Marita Nordhaug

Loss, Dying and Bereavement in the Criminal Justice System
Edited by Sue Read, Sotirios Santatzoglou and Anthony Wrigley

Professional Identity in the Caring Professions
Meaning, Measurement and Mastery
Edited by Roger Ellis and Elaine Hogard

Trade Union Strategies and Healthcare Marketization
Jennie Auffenberg

Leadership at the Intersection of Gender and Race in Healthcare and Science
Case Studies and Tools
Edited by Danielle Laraque-Arena, Lauren Germain, Virginia Young and Rivers Laraque-Ho

Exploring End of Life Experience
Facing Death
Dr Helen Besemeres

Understanding the Grief and Loss Experiences of Carers
Research, Practitioner and Personal Perspectives
Edited by Joanna Horne and Kerry Jones

For more information about this series, please visit: www.routledge.com/Routledge-Key-Themes-in-Health-and-Society/book-series/RKTHS

Understanding the Grief and Loss Experiences of Carers

Research, Practitioner and Personal Perspectives

Edited by Kerry Jones and Joanna Horne

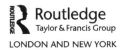

LONDON AND NEW YORK

First published 2025
by Routledge
4 Park Square, Milton Park, Abingdon, Oxon OX14 4RN

and by Routledge
605 Third Avenue, New York, NY 10158

Routledge is an imprint of the Taylor & Francis Group, an informa business

© 2025 selection and editorial matter, Joanna Horne and Kery Jones;
individual chapters, the contributors

The right of Joanna Horne and Kery Jones to be identified as the authors
of the editorial material, and of the authors for their individual chapters,
has been asserted in accordance with sections 77 and 78 of the Copyright,
Designs and Patents Act 1988.

All rights reserved. No part of this book may be reprinted or reproduced or
utilised in any form or by any electronic, mechanical, or other means, now
known or hereafter invented, including photocopying and recording, or in
any information storage or retrieval system, without permission in writing
from the publishers.

Trademark notice: Product or corporate names may be trademarks or
registered trademarks, and are used only for identification and explanation
without intent to infringe.

British Library Cataloguing-in-Publication Data
A catalogue record for this book is available from the British Library

Library of Congress Cataloging-in-Publication Data
Names: Jones, Kerry (College teacher), editor. | Horne, Joanna, editor.
Title: Understanding the grief and loss experiences of carers : research,
    practitioner and personal perspectives / edited by Kerry Jones and
    Joanna Horne.
Description: Abingdon, Oxon ; New York, NY : Routledge, 2024. | Includes
    bibliographical references and index.
Identifiers: LCCN 2024018371 (print) | LCCN 2024018372 (ebook) | ISBN
    9781032564043 (hardback) | ISBN 9781032566009 (paperback) | ISBN
    9781003435365 (ebook)
Subjects: LCSH: Grief. | Loss (Psychology) | Caregivers—Psychology.
Classification: LCC BF575.G7 U5248 2024 (print) | LCC BF575.G7
    (ebook) | DDC 362/.0425—dc23/eng/20240609
LC record available at https://lccn.loc.gov/2024018371
LC ebook record available at https://lccn.loc.gov/2024018372

ISBN: 9781032564043 (hbk)
ISBN: 9781032566009 (pbk)
ISBN: 9781003435365 (ebk)

DOI: 10.4324/9781003435365

Typeset in Times New Roman
by Apex CoVantage, LLC

Contents

List of figures and tables	*vii*
List of contributors	*viii*
Introduction	*xii*
KERRY JONES AND JOANNA HORNE	

1 Ambiguous loss: Personal and professional reflections   1
ANDREA PERRY

2 Impact on identity for those working as healthcare professionals when taking on the role of carer   15
JULIE MESSENGER

3 'I could cry all day, every day, about my losses': Caring for young adults with life-shortening conditions – families' experiences of disruption and loss   27
SARAH EARLE, MADDIE BLACKBURN, LIZZIE CHAMBERS, JULIA DOWNING, KATE FLEMMING, JAMIE HALE, HANNAH R. MARSTON, LINDSAY O'DELL, VALERIE SINASON AND SALLY WHITNEY

4 From physically active to physically inactive: Understanding the experiences of a familial carer's loss of self   41
NICHOLA KENTZER, MARTIN PENSON AND MELINDA SPENCER

5 Both sides of the coin: A mother's experience of caring for an adult daughter living with serious life-limiting illness   54
SUSAN WALKER

vi *Contents*

6 'God hasn't given up on them': Christian dementia carers'
  narratives of experiencing and challenging 'anticipatory
  grief' and 'social death'   65
  JENNIFER RILEY AND JOHN SWINTON

7 The grief of care partners of people living and dying with
  dementia: A psychodynamic perspective   79
  PHIL MCEVOY, ESTHER RAMSAY-JONES, AMANDA BARRELL,
  RACHEL YATES-HOYLES AND EMMA SMITH

8 When an adult with significant caregiving responsibilities
  for children is at end-of-life with cancer: A carer's
  pre-bereavement and post-bereavement experiences   94
  JEFFREY R. HANNA, CHERITH J. SEMPLE, LISA STRUTT

9 When caring ends: Exploring the hidden aspects of loss in
  trajectories out of caring in Australia   110
  EMMA KIRBY, GISELLE NEWTON, LOUISA SMITH, IVA STRNADOVÁ,
  BRENDAN CHURCHILL, LUKAS HOFFSTÄTTER, SARAH JUDD-LAM,
  AND CHRISTY E. NEWMAN

10 Former carers: Grief, loss and other stories   123
  MARY LARKIN AND ALISOUN MILNE

  Index   *135*

Figures and tables

Figures

4.1   Socioecological model of the barriers and facilitators to carers'
physical activity   43

Tables

3.1   Inclusion and exclusion criteria   29
6.1   Frequency of denominations of TEIs at which participants worked   67
6.2   Frequency of locations of TEIs at which participants worked   68

Contributors

Amanda Barrell is a British Association for Counselling and Psychotherapy registered counsellor and Empowered Carers Facilitator for Age UK Salford, providing talking therapies for family care partners of people living with a dementia.

Maddie Blackburn is a retired solicitor, former CEO of a hospice and a National Charity's Care Director. With Professor Sarah Earle, she co-edited *Sex, intimacy and living with life-shortening conditions* (2024). She completed her doctorate and other post-doctoral research with Professor Earle at The Open University.

Lizzie Chambers is Programmes Manager for the International Children's Palliative Care Network, UK. Lizzie has worked in children's palliative care for 21 years, as Chief Executive of ACT and then Director of Programmes at Together for Short Lives, where she authored many of the charity's publications and led various national programmes.

Brendan Churchill is an Australian Research Council DECRA Senior Research Fellow in Sociology at The University of Melbourne, Australia.

Julia Downing is the Chief Executive of the International Children's Palliative Care Network, UK/Uganda. She is an experienced palliative care nurse, educationalist and researcher. Julia is a professor at universities in Uganda, Serbia and the UK. She has worked within palliative care for 30 years, with 20 of those working internationally in Uganda, Africa, Eastern Europe and globally.

Sarah Earle is Professor of Social Science at Nottingham Trent University, UK. She is a medical sociologist with international expertise in the sociology of disability, human reproduction and sexual health. She has published widely in these fields.

Kate Flemming works in the Department of Health Sciences, University of York, UK. She has a clinical background in palliative care nursing and her research concentrates on equity of access to palliative care. Kate is a co-convenor of the international Cochrane Qualitative and Implementation Methods Group.

Contributors ix

Jamie Hale is an independent researcher based in the UK, with lived experience of life-limiting and life-threatening conditions, and an interest in co-production in health and disability research. They are CEO of Pathfinders Neuromuscular Alliance.

Jeffrey R. Hanna is a Lecturer in Clinical Cancer Nursing at Ulster University and South Eastern Health and Social Care Trust, Northern Ireland. In his clinical role, Jeffrey is passionate about the provision of psycho-social and supportive care to patients, carers and families impacted by cancer. Jeffrey's key research interests are family-centred cancer care and promoting healthcare and patient education in cancer care through digital technology.

Lukas Hoffstätter is Senior Research and Development Officer at Carers NSW, Australia.

Sarah Judd-Lam is Executive Manager, Policy, Development and Research, at Carers NSW, Australia.

Nichola Kentzer is a Senior Lecturer in Sport, Exercise and Coaching at The Open University, UK. Nichola, a HCPC registered Practitioner Psychologist (Sport and Exercise) and carer herself, focuses her research on understanding mechanisms to support carer wellbeing, including physical activity and learning.

Emma Kirby is Professor of Sociology in the Faculty of Arts, Design & Architecture at UNSW, Sydney, Australia.

Mary Larkin is Professor of care, carers and caring at the Open University, UK. She has extensive experience of carer research and working with carers organisations. Mary has published widely and been involved in many local, national and international bodies, committees and commissions. She has developed courses about and for carers as well as initiatives to support staff and students who are carers.

Hannah R. Marston is a Research Fellow at The Open University, UK. She conducts inter-and-cross disciplinary research in the fields of digital technologies and practices, gerontology, health, age-friendly cities and communities; and has published a wide breadth on these topics. Hannah collaborates with international colleagues on several projects and her research has been cited in several policy documents.

Phil McEvoy is a psychodynamic psychotherapist. He is an Empowered Carers Facilitator for Age UK, Salford, and supervises weekly reflective practice sessions for the team.

Julie Messenger is a registered nurse, working as a nurse academic at The Open University, UK. Julie has held a number of senior roles in nursing practice and academic leadership, including work for the Professional Regulatory Body for UK Nursing, the Nursing and Midwifery Council as a quality assurance reviewer and as a Lead Reviewer for the Office for Students, England.

x *Contributors*

Alisoun Milne is Professor Emerita of Social Gerontology and Social Work at the University of Kent, UK. She has been involved in work on family caring for over twenty years; this included being a member of the independent advisory committee, the Standing Commission on Carers. Alisoun has written widely on care and caring issues and is embedded in national and international care related research and practice networks.

Christy E. Newman is a Professor in the Centre for Social Research in Health, and Deputy Dean Research in the Faculty of Arts, Design & Architecture at UNSW, Sydney, Australia.

Giselle Newton is a Postdoctoral Research Fellow in the Centre for Digital Cultures and Societies at the University of Queensland, Australia.

Lindsay O'Dell is Professor of Critical Developmental Psychology at The Open University, UK. Her research has a focus on disability, neurodiversity and long-term health conditions.

Martin Penson is a former UK secondary school physical education teacher, and former familial carer for his mum. In addition to his sport science degree and teaching qualifications, he is educated at postgraduate level in physical activity and public health.

Andrea Perry is an integrative psychotherapist in the UK, specialising in attachment, loss and trauma, a former Chair of the British Association of Dramatherapists, author and trainer. She worked within the International Family Tracing Service and Psychosocial and Mental Health Team of the British Red Cross for 14 years and was a carer for both parents.

Esther Ramsay-Jones is a psychodynamic psychotherapist and practitioner-researcher. She is a lecturer at Birkbeck Centre for Counselling and has published work on the relational field of dementia and palliative care.

Jennifer Riley is Research Fellow in Divinity and Religious Studies at the University of Aberdeen, Scotland, UK. Her research explores religion and theology as they intersect with deathcare and healthcare.

Valerie Sinason is a UK writer and psychoanalyst. She is President of the Institute of Psychotherapy and Disability and on the Board of the International Society of Trauma and Dissociation. Founder of the clinic for Dissociative Studies and a former Consultant Psychoanalyst at the Tavistock Clinic and St George's Hospital, she has written and published over 25 Books and 400 papers. She received the BPS award for innovation excellence and the ISSTD Lifetime Achievement Award.

Cherith J. Semple is a Professor of Clinical Cancer Nursing at Ulster University and South Eastern Health and Social Care Trust. As a clinical academic, Cherith has extensive experience in oncology nursing and has led the Family-centred Cancer Care programme of work at Ulster University's Institute of Nursing and Health Research for almost 15 years, having published and presented widely on the topic of parental cancer.

Emma Smith is Project Manager for The Empowered Conversations Approach, Age UK Salford, delivering communication courses, one-to-one dementia-focused therapeutic support and regular groups and webinars for professionals and families affected by dementia.

Louisa Smith is a Senior Lecturer in the Discipline of Disability and Inclusion, Faculty of Health, Deakin University, Australia.

Melinda Spencer is a senior lecturer in BSc Health Sciences at the University of Northampton, UK. Melinda is an active researcher specialising in qualitative experiential research and evaluation. Projects include family relationships and transitions, social prescription impact and outcomes and, the impact of creative and community dance on older adults.

Iva Strnadová is a Professor in Special Education and Disability Studies at UNSW Sydney, Australia. She is also the Academic Research Lead at the Disability Innovation Institute at UNSW.

Lisa Strutt is an accredited professional Leadership Coach (ICF) specialising in transition and runs her own coaching practice. She's interested in the science of coaching and is a Fellow of the Institute of Coaching (Harvard McLean Medical School). She was carer to her late husband, John, who died of pancreatic cancer in 2020, is a Trustee of Northern Ireland Pancreatic Cancer Charity (NIPANC) and bereaved mum who advocates for better conversations about death and dying.

John Swinton is Professor in Practical Theology and Pastoral Care at the University of Aberdeen, Scotland, UK. He is a former mental health nurse and has published widely within the area of mental health, disability and dementia.

Susan Walker is an informal carer. She is an ordained Christian minister in the North-East of England, UK, and a former hospice chaplain. She writes about death and dying and has authored two books from Christian perspectives and written several academic healthcare articles, focusing on the perspectives of terminally ill people and their carers.

Rachel Yates-Hoyles is an accredited coach and mentor who worked as Empowered Carers Project Manager for 5 years at Age UK, Salford where she remains a member of the steering group team.

Introduction

Kerry Jones and Joanna Horne

Carers provide unpaid care to family members or friends requiring support due to illness, disability, mental health difficulties or addiction. As this caring role is informal and generally unrecorded, there are no precise figures for the number of carers internationally. However, based on estimates that are available in individual countries, it would be reasonable to expect that between 12 and 20 percent of the population worldwide are providing unpaid care to family members or friends.

Whether care provided is related to a long-term or life-limiting condition, many carers experience a multitude of losses including indefinite loss characterised by biographical disruption. Carers may also experience ambiguous loss, such as a loss of an emotional connection, or anticipatory grief, as multiple losses such as companionship, personal freedom, and control manifest. While many carers are dedicated and committed to their role, they are subject to burnout and disenfranchised grief. That is a grief which is not acknowledged or recognised. When the role of caregiver ends, due to the death of those cared for, this can represent a major change and a period of significant adjustment for carers, leading to a range of emotions experienced in the form of loneliness, sadness, lacking in purpose, and resentment for the things that have been missed. Caregiving can also be life-affirming for some, and, in some instances, carers may experience relief or calmness when care responsibilities cease.

Caring for people experiencing loss is an integral part of being a caregiver, but also features in the work of helping professions, whether it is explicitly part of their work such as in counselling, or implicit as in social work, nursing, teaching, medicine, community and voluntary work.

This interdisciplinary and interprofessional edited collection brings together authors from a wide range of backgrounds in research, teaching and professional practice, many with personal experiences of loss that have informed their thinking and practice, as well as coping in terms of resilience and self-preservation. The collection increases our understanding of carers' experience of loss, by drawing carers' experiences across the life course (younger and older carers) together, and at the same time contributing to improving support services for carers prior to and following the death of a person cared for.

The chapters in the collection are diverse in both focus and format, including theoretical contributions and psychodynamic perspectives, reports of research

Introduction xiii

findings, and a wealth of personal accounts, with many chapters interweaving the voice of the carer with the academic or professional perspective. The kinds of experiences discussed include transitioning through the caregiving experience such as finding meaning, reconstructing identity and daily life, coping with familial expectations and developing resilience, and encompass caring for others at all stages of the life course. Although the primary focus is on the ways in which the experience of loss is framed by caregiving, a diversity of experience in terms of social class, age, ethnicity, culture and religion is also represented in the book.

The chapters

In the first chapter by Andrea Perry, ambiguous loss is foregrounded by the author's personal account of caregiving for elderly parents and, second, through the author's lens as a psychotherapist supporting carers as part of her professional practice. Turning to Boss' framework to understand ambiguous loss, the chapter provides a way to comprehend some of the ways carers confront uncertainty and, in turn, how they can be supported to transcend the impact by revising their attachment and identity to the person they care for. Through this lens, carers can begin to find ways to reconstruct their identity positively and, with it, discover new hope.

In keeping with the theme of the personal and professional, the next chapter by Julie Messenger considers the impact for those working as a health care professional while taking on the role of a care provider of a spouse. Reflecting on these experiences, Messenger provides insight into the dilemmas inherent in occupying two roles. The chapter describes a sustained trajectory of caregiving which involves taking on the role of advocate, on the one hand, and holding privileged knowledge as a nurse while negotiating for care interventions to improve the health of her husband on the other. As Messenger poignantly recounts, loss as experienced by herself as a carer and by her husband as a care recipient are varied yet provide much needed insight on the importance of empowering recipients of care in decision making.

Turning to the care of young adults with life-shortening conditions, Chapter 3, by Sarah Earle and colleagues, focuses on family carers' experiences of biographical disruption and anticipatory loss. The chapter provides a much-needed focus on a widely neglected issue in the literature which concerns the 'new population' of young people with life-shortening conditions who were not expected to live yet, due to advances in medical treatment, are living longer than in previous years. Based on co-produced research undertaken during the COVID-19 pandemic, the consequences of lockdown and shielding are discussed. From these narrations you get to hear about the prevailing idealised discourse about babies and parenthood that does little to prepare parents for the loss of a potential future as a family and of the anticipatory loss of their young person.

Chapter 4, by Nichola Kentzer and colleagues, presents a further research study which focuses on carers' experiences of the loss of sense of self brought about by the loss of physical activity. Physical activity is a vital health benefit for many carers yet, as studies suggest, multiple barriers exist which can prevent carers who xiv *K. Jones and J. Horne*

previously engaged from doing so. Told from the perspective of a carer who was a participant as well as a co-researcher in the study, the chapter reflects on barriers such as guilt, time, and fatigue and how this impacted on his loss of athletic identity.

In the fifth chapter, Susan Walker provides a personal account of caring for an adult daughter with a life-limiting condition. Biographical disruption and trajectory features as the central narrative, in which Walker discusses loss in terms of paid employment, independent housing and the ability to make plans for the future. Such losses, Walker reflects, are not acknowledged socially, leading to disenfranchised grief. The trajectory of care is also considered beyond losses through the lens of reconstruction theory and the dual process model of grieving to also describe a care experience which is life-affirming. Here are two adults, a mother and daughter who share a life together and, since diagnosis of a life-limiting condition, have found meaning, a sense of purpose and even privilege. Chapter 6 by Jennifer Riley and John Swinton brings our attention to theology and faith in the context of dementia. Based on research undertaken with people living with dementia, their carers and theological educators, the findings highlight the challenges in overcoming ideas about social and spiritual death, such that people with dementia are perceived to be no longer socially or spiritually connected. Such notions, as perceived by participants of the study, are unhelpful, culminating as they do in disenfranchisement and disempowerment for the carer and person experiencing dementia. The authors proffer a supportive and practical outcome which requires the church to respond caringly. That is, to acknowledge the pain of loss and grief while also affirming the value agency and social significance of the carer and the person experiencing dementia.

Continuing with the theme of dementia, Phil McEvoy and colleagues consider carer grief from a psychodynamic perspective in Chapter 7. Carers interviewed as part of the authors' research, in keeping with the experiences of many carers, attest to the presence of powerful internal conflicts which describe a caring role which is rewarding yet impacts on one's ability to mourn. Anticipatory grief, ambiguous loss and disenfranchisement are central to participants' experiences while in their caring role and following the death of the person with dementia. The chapter demonstrates the value of psychodynamic counselling, which can benefit carers by giving an emotional space to talk, and ways in which counsellors can provide professional support for care partners to deal with pre-death and post-death experiences.

Chapter 8 by Jeffrey Hanna and colleagues brings the focus of caring in the context of pre- and post-bereavement experiences. Presented in two parts, the first part focuses on a carer's experience of preparing children for the death of an adult, who has a significant caregiving responsibility for them, from cancer. The second part focuses on the role of supporting and caring for children following the death of an adult. What follows is an in-depth account of living with uncertainties such as how and when to share the prognosis with the children and prepare them for an impending death of a parent and how to cope with one's own grief and those of the children post-death. In so doing, the chapter provides insight on ways in which to support carers in a similar situation and also evidence-based recommendations for professionals to support a carer throughout an end-of-life experience and beyond.

Introduction xv

In the final two chapters, the focus is on former carers with research involving focus groups undertaken by Emma Kirby and colleagues in Australia and case studies research undertaken by Mary Larkin and Alisoun Milne in the UK. Both studies explore the often-hidden aspects of loss experienced by carers transitioning out of their caring role over the life course as 'serial' carers. Yet each care trajectory, as the authors in Chapters 9 and 10 argue, represents the loss of a caring role in each transition and, with it, grief responses such as distress, negative feelings such as anger and a loss of self-esteem. Both chapters provide much-needed insight into the multiple challenges carers experience which include, but are not limited to, a loss of identity, and a loss of sense of self and purpose as carers navigate life beyond caring and one in which financial precarity and vulnerability may prevail. Such experiences as depicted in these chapters are often rendered invisible and disenfranchised by the social milieu to which carers relate. The authors make a vital case for a need for policy to re-think conceptual deficits as well as the need for the improved provision of support for former carers.

1 Ambiguous loss
Personal and professional reflections

Andrea Perry

Introduction

This chapter draws on personal and professional perspectives. I first provide an overview of ambiguous loss (Boss, 2000, 2007, 2016) and some of its structural and psychological impacts on carers (Dupuis, 2002), mindful that those we care for are likely experiencing it too (beyond the scope of this brief chapter). I will share some of my own experiences as a carer of elderly parents, alongside those of other adult carers (names and details have been changed), who have also experienced the impact of ambiguous loss on their lives and their families. I will, on occasion, use '*we*' and '*our*' to imply my shared experience with other carers. The small sample of participants providing narrative were, like myself, all professional women in middle age, of diverse ethnicities, with long-term caring responsibilities for elderly parents. Each participant was invited to reflect on their experience in relation to a summary of ambiguous loss theory, including the impact on them and what they found helped them manage. Each discussion was held individually, and space and time was given to the emotional impact of discussing ambiguous loss.

Impact of ambiguous loss

The impacts of ambiguous loss (adapted from Boss, 2000, 2007; Dupuis, 2002; Perry, 2016; Knight and Glitterman, 2019; Nathanson and Rogers, 2020) include both structural and psychological effects. Structural impact may include decision-making difficulties, ambivalence (about the person being cared for or the situation), internal conflict, preoccupation and isolation, confusion, self-neglect, sense of being in limbo or paralysed, powerlessness and the avoidance of, or indifference to, ordinary rituals, roles and celebrations. Psychological impacts may include depression, hopelessness and suicidal ideation, panic and anxiety, guilt, shame, feeling of being robbed, aggression, addiction, tension, stress, traumatisation, stress-related illness, and somatisation.

To develop resilience in response to ambiguous loss, Boss (2016, p. 273), updating her earlier guidance, suggests supporting individuals through:

1. finding meaning
2. adjusting mastery

DOI: 10.4324/9781003435365-1

2 A. Perry

3. reconstructing identity
4. normalising ambivalence
5. revising attachment
6. discovering new hope.

Nathanson and Rogers (2020) expand on these to include learning about the grief trajectory, whilst Hirsch (2022) stresses allowing multiple truths about carers' changing experience to co-exist (i.e., developing both/and thinking, rather than either/or thinking), and seeking professional help to manage.

Carers and ambiguous loss

The experiences of the participants interviewed for this chapter will be used to explore Boss' key principles for enabling people to work through ambiguous loss, towards finding hope and meaning. Each person's diverse needs, background, gender, age, race, sexuality, culture, history, role and experience will mean that no two pathways are the same, though there may be commonalities. In understanding that it is the situation of ambiguous loss in which we find ourselves that is abnormal, and not our very human responses, we may find some measure of peace and the strength to change what we can, perhaps the capacity to tolerate what we cannot change, plus the ability to work out the difference. The German word for fortitude is *langmut* – literally, long courage – what is surely needed here.

None of the carers interviewed for this chapter encountered a professional working with their parents who was also specifically tasked to work therapeutically with their loss and grief as carers. The carers met professionals only when their parent was being supported, treated, assessed, rushed into hospital, and so on, as did I. However, given the significance of the carer's role, it is essential that our needs are taken into account, and neither glossed over (for example, with glib comments like 'You carers are all wonderful') nor neglected, because to do so not only has impact on the carer, but also knock-on impact on the one being cared for, our parent.

Professionals, too, may be triggered by ambiguous loss (see below). So, in conclusion, I will highlight how professionals might provide carers with brief moments of psychosocial support, stabilising validation and empathy, to help carers build tolerance of the ambiguity they are facing and find creative ways to live with it. Such knowledge may be helpful for professionals who wish to support carers when they encounter them, whilst providing treatment or care for an elderly patient (the carer's parent).

Learning ambiguous loss from the inside – a personal account

As a psychosocial practitioner for an international charity, with a background as a psychotherapist, I first came across the concept of ambiguous loss (Boss, 2000) and the work of Pauline Boss in 2013, in my role supporting people looking for missing family members. Their loss of those beloved people was ambiguous – they didn't

Ambiguous loss 3

know what had become of them, whether they lived or had died. In addition, they experienced multiple other ambiguous losses in lives characterised by systemic and global uncertainty. Working with such families for eight years, using the British Red Cross psychosocial model, CALMER (Davidson et al., 2022) I expanded my understanding of loss and grief as taught on professional training courses (such as my disciplines of psychotherapy and dramatherapy as well as within counselling, social work, psychology, medicine, nursing, social care etc) and supported clients towards developing lives – or moments – of hope and purpose alongside the yearning for news, any news, of their family.

It took a long time for me to transfer my professional understanding of ambiguous loss to my personal circumstances, where I was involved with caring for my father, who had vascular dementia, and, after his death, my mother, who had two physical conditions worsening in tandem. Once I made the connection, I recognised the multiplicity of ambiguous losses which being a carer of elderly parents may involve (Dupuis, 2002; Nathanson and Rogers, 2020), to which I and my siblings were subjected. Our parents' capacities deteriorated, returned, deteriorated again with a change of medication, or rallied against the odds, an exhausting switchback ride that sometimes seemed as if it would keep my father, and then my mother, going longer than we 'children' alongside them.

I experienced many of the impacts described by Boss (2016) which I had witnessed amongst my clients separated from their families: the sense of being in limbo, powerless, unable to concentrate or make decisions, together with guilt, shame, sadness, the feeling of being robbed, and tremendous tension. There were occasions when I found myself raging out loud whilst out walking, so great was the tension and intense sense of being stuck.

To work through the ambiguous losses to the point where I could, some of the time, find peace and a degree of 'mastery' in the moment (Boss, 2016), and give up trying to control the rest, took a long time, alongside much personal reflection, self-forgiveness and support from other carers, friends, and family. The calm, kind presence of one hospice nurse who genuinely listened and assured me with sincerity that my experience was natural, under the circumstances, was a rare and welcome professional contribution.

Having learnt about Boss' principles for learning to tolerate ambiguous loss, I recognised them in action within my own experience. For example, towards the end of her life in the family home, I arrived to find my mother, now alone and missing my father, in very low spirits, fretful, woebegone and distressed, suffering from increasing physical pain and exhaustion. The room was cluttered and untidy, the bathroom a mess. There was nothing I could do about her pain, nor her sadness, nor about the concern that another hospital admission might be imminent ('adjusting mastery'; Boss, 2016). But I could wipe, clean, sort papers, polish furniture and the family photos, bring in bright flowers from the garden ('reconstruct identity', ibid.). In the room, returned to freshness and peaceful order in that lovely, quiet moment after a hoover is turned off, we had tea and slices of Victoria sponge made to her special recipe for family occasions, on her pretty plates ('revising attachments', ibid.). And the sun came out. She thanked me, simply, and sighed, deeply;

4 *A. Perry*

restored for that little time together, I think, not to any stable state, but just for that moment, to a small and precious sense of feeling safe, content, and loved; as was I ('finding meaning', 'discovering hope', ibid.).

I return to such treasured memories often, now that my parents are gone. There are many other stories, some harrowing, traumatic and deeply sad, some shaming and frustrating, some repetitive and boring. But I hold moments such as these, in which we jointly honoured what there was and who we were together, whilst equally honouring what and who had been lost, as symbols of something deeply precious, hard won (Boss, 2000). To me they are emblematic of what is possible within ambiguous loss; finding something real, grounded, hopeful and even joyful, at the same time as grief, as hopelessness, as not knowing (Mannix, 2018). There is no quick fix; learning to tolerate ambiguous loss takes time, understanding, connection with others and courage. Nor is it a one-way journey, any more than is any other kind of grief.

The journey of ambiguous loss and its impact

The concept of ambiguous loss was described by Dr Pauline Boss (2000) as the experience of an ongoing loss characterised by uncertainty. We may continually ask ourselves: Is this loss permanent, or is it retrievable? How do I have a life and find meaning whilst not knowing?

When children or adults go missing, however temporarily, whatever the cause, watching at a distance, we can viscerally understand the pain of enduring the loss: initial terror and disbelief turning to a frozen state of limbo and preoccupation with getting any kind of news, first with hope and, increasingly, whilst the world moves on, with despair (Tahmazian, 2015).

This is ambiguous loss. Its profile (Boss, 2000, 2007, 2016; Dupuis, 2002; Knight and Glitterman, 2019; Nathanson and Rogers, 2020) contrasts in many ways with the impact of what we might term finite loss, a once-and-for-all loss, like a death, with its more familiar patterns of non-linear recovery from grief, complex and otherwise, alongside varying rituals, and the possibility of varying degrees of 'closure' whilst continuing attachments in different forms.

However, ambiguous loss is not only about an individual being physically absent or missing, it can also be losing connection with a person as we once knew them. With Alzheimer's or dementia or other long term degenerative conditions (Dupuis, 2002), the parents of carers may still be their core selves, but they may be in an altered state of mind and faculty. Thus, the relationship we had together, and the memories we held in common, are 'there, but not there' (Boss, 2007, p. 105). Ambiguous loss also includes loss of identity, confidence, working roles, a social life, hope, and much besides. Carers themselves may lose touch with aspects of selves and their lives, unclear whether they will ever return, or whether they, or the people they are caring for, have changed irrevocably (ibid.).

A carer's experience of ambiguous loss may start with a traumatic, one-off event. For example, a road traffic accident or a stroke leaves a family member in a physical state from which their relatives – and/or that individual – cannot know if they will return. Alternatively, ambiguous loss may only become apparent over

Ambiguous loss 5

time. There may be confusing reversals, a 'switchback ride'. Parents with Alzheimer's, dementia, Parkinson's, and degenerative conditions of genetic, or other origin with a slow unsteady onset may appear to have lost faculties; but one morning, carers may be met with an apparent return of capacity, and an indignant refusal to allow them to give the care that was so essential and appreciated the day before.

Throughout the progress of the condition, adult carers, alongside the person who is unwell and other family members, enter the turbulent journey of chronic ambiguous loss, for which they may feel unprepared. Hazel, one of the women interviewed for this chapter, encountered an important and painful new phase of the journey. Hazel's mother from London's working-class East End, who used to describe herself as 'poor, proud and particular', had been, before her stroke, a fiercely independent woman. Hazel felt highly anxious about what would happen to her relationship with her mother when she and her siblings had to take over aspects of her mother's care, knowing she would hate it. Having to step in to take charge presented Hazel with some of the impacts of ambiguous loss, those of grieving for her 'fiercely independent' mother whilst her mother is still alive, as well as the uncertainty of taking on the new responsibility, not at all sure their relationship would survive the change in responsibility.

Rowan is one of two siblings caring for their mother who has dementia, their father having died with dementia during the pandemic:

> I'd say I feel I can't get on with the next stage of my life, even down to where I live; I don't feel settled, you need to feel settled so you can think and organise, or be creative and I just can't; you like to tick things off, from a list, don't you? But it's too exhausting . . . It's like being in limbo, in a big fog, you know there are rocks and scree to the side of the path, and probably a drop, but you can't see them. I feel like, just let me have my little life.

Rowan's experience highlights how ambiguous losses involved in the caring role can make carers feel as if their own lives are on hold – yet they keep on living, even when feeling compromised. They may experience ambiguous loss of roles they had until then: opportunities, finances, dreams, relationships, a sense of self-worth, self-esteem, trust in the world as a safe, fair and just place where working hard and doing the right thing should, they might have formerly believed, lead to good results, the right outcome (Boss, 2000; Dupuis, 2002; Tahmazian, 2015). There is a sense of the ambiguous loss of control, of being able to predict, plan, have a firm basis for making decisions and confidence in their ability to follow them through, an isolating loss of hope, and possibly the loss of their own mental and physical wellbeing.

Rowan's formerly capable, confident mother now anxiously calls her, day and night, sometimes 12 or 13 times in 24 hours; calls can be up to 20 minutes, often going over the same ground:

> Different emotions are running through your head all the time. It just feels never-ending, I feel trapped, useless, tearful, it's frustrating; there's guilt; I should be happy to do this, and I am, but when [her mother rings again],

6   *A. Perry*

it's tempting to ignore it . . . but it might be *that* call, saying 'Come now'. Sometimes my heart pounds, I feel like I'm on a knife edge. Even when she was with my brother for a day, I kept checking my phone.

As carers, we can feel like Sisyphus, pushing the same boulder uphill every day, perhaps neglecting ourselves, wondering how long this will continue. Sometimes we wish it would end, so that we can be relieved and start to grieve properly, resolve the ambiguity; sometimes hating ourselves for wishing that, and needing to forgive ourselves for our thoughts, if we can. Or we may want to postpone the final goodbye for as long as possible, forever. We are grieving for the person we care about at the same times as caring for them, for the absence of someone we love, in their very presence.

This is especially so if the person being cared for behaves in new and uncharacteristic ways. Lonely and feeling lost, but bound to a stranger, we yearn for who we both were. In her 'joint story of me and my mother', Caoimhe, a long-term carer for her mother, sees herself as someone who enjoyed her life, an optimistic person, but now finds it difficult to have a sense of that self much of the time. She questions whether her mother 'is ever going to come back – is she going to get better?'. She experienced her mother as a 'challenging character to grow up around', and that it 'wasn't all sunny days', but now recognises 'multiple layers of loss' around her of the early relationship, where her mother was 'the strong protector, the safe place for me, the person who would sing to me and love me'. Her mother can be 'quite vile' to her now, as she rages against the injustice of her life and 'rages at me, for want of anyone better'. As her mother goes 'in and out of herself', Caoimhe, who feels paralysed, unable to focus or plan, and having strong palpitations, is left questioning 'Is the mother I love there anymore? Do I even love her anymore?'.

Ambivalent feelings we had for the individual affect how we provide care in the moment, and our feelings about needing or choosing to do so. There may be guilt, resentment, and shame that we are not able to live up to our own unattainable standards of what we imagine a carer 'should' be feeling. Unless, and until, we can find a way to tolerate the ambiguous nature of our losses, we are subject to their frozen, preoccupying, paralysing, hope-undermining impact. We feel overwhelmed, out of control, in a heightened state of tension and agitation, anxiety and potentially depression (Dupuis, 2002). Our capacity to care may become blocked (Hughes and Baylin, 2012), reduced to grim determination by isolation and the apparent lack of meaning in what we are repeatedly having to do, when there is little or no reciprocity, or external empathy for, or validation of, our experience. Rowan comments on how her changing responses to her mother bring her further struggles:

And I think my sense of humour has gone a bit: when my energy is low, if she's called me at night, all the little pecking [of repeated calls] all day . . . and these days you can see who it is, on your phone, which makes it worse . . . then I get impatient, but Mum doesn't need that, which brings back another big dollop of guilt, with double guilt on the side.

Ambiguous loss 7

Other strong emotions impact carers, sometimes unexpectedly. Caoimhe's mother was someone 'people used to admire'; her verbal attacks on Caoimhe can now be so venomous that professionals have expressed concern for Caoimhe. With incredible strength and generosity, she recognises her ambivalent feelings:

> I can feel the solidarity that people feel for me about her, but then I feel shame for [my mother], and a bit ashamed of myself that I'm glad of the solidarity – I feel sad for her because she was better than that – it's hard – I feel so sorry for her.

Often feeling intensely isolated, having to give up some of her work in order to manage her energy for her caring role, Caoimhe has lost multiple safe harbours, not only within the family, but also of work and the wider social setting of community. Professionals see one person; carers experience the painful ambiguity of having both the sense of their parent as they were, whom they grieve, alongside who they seem to be now.

My experience reflects something of Caoimhe's sense of disorientation. In the last few weeks of my father's life, I found the casual indifference of some nursing staff to the state my father was left in almost unbearable, and very isolating. He had always been impeccably turned out, smelling freshly of toothpaste, polished shoes and Imperial Leather soap, now left helpless in messy bedsheets with his pyjamas all awry. It was heart-breaking to see this frail, yet still courteous man, in such need, talked over, marginalised, treated as a task someone would get round to when they chose, rather than respected as the committed, playful, contradictory and tender-hearted man of great courage I could still see and missed deeply, still himself at core. Speechless with grief, I put newspaper cuttings of his activities as a WWII boy scout working at the hospital in a frame beside his bed, almost forcing any professional who stopped for a moment to look at it, my way to honour who he really was, or had been.

There are no rituals to help us come to terms with what is happening and limited public recognition. Until we can identify and understand what we are going through, our grief remains disenfranchised (Knight and Glitterman, 2019); one which does not simply fear to speak its name but doesn't actually know what that name is.

Polarisation

A common response to ambiguous loss is to polarise, to fall into either/or thinking, perhaps a means of managing anxiety stirred up by uncertainty (Dupuis, 2002). For example, different members of Hazel's family took polarised positions about their mother's capacity: 'Our mother is just having a temporary wobble about sleeping upstairs, she's fine', versus 'She can't sleep upstairs anymore, it's too dangerous'. The carers interviewed reported some family members wanting immediate action and to take control, whereas others found their decision-making ability eroded,

8   *A. Perry*

leaving them feeling marginalised. Contrasting views, based on an individual's own experience, perspective, habitual methods of coping and personal style, usual role in the family and so on, can add tensions and rifts to the already stressful family pot. On some occasions, as with Hazel and her family, a whole family may swing into action on a surge of anxiety, only to regret decisions when events pan out differently to their worst fears. Hazel and her brother rushed a stairlift into their mother's house after her stroke, never really knowing if it would be used. In fact, their mother died only a few weeks later, and it wasn't. Hazel feels the hospital professionals had pressed for action, to free up her bed; no-one suggested a more reflective approach to managing the uncertainties.

Foreclosing on discussions to change things to quickly create 'resolution' helps a family avoid the tension of loss and uncertainty, but a more relational, reflective, discursive and adaptive approach helps them begin to tolerate ambiguity and arrive at more inclusive, considered decisions. From a psychosocial perspective (Tahmazian, 2015; Davidson et al., 2022), professionals equally need to be mindful of the impact of ambiguity on a family's capacity to hear, reflect and think clearly, and indeed recognise that they too may be tempted to defend against uncertainty by moving prematurely into action. Professionals also need to consider the impact of changing layers of the social context in which care is happening, including global events such as a pandemic, as a key component in helping carers understand their experience, and choose action in the interests of their physical, mental, emotional and relational health.

Integrating Boss' principles for developing tolerance of ambiguous loss into reality

Acknowledging our mixed feelings and emotions as carers, and knowing they are natural, is best summed up by Rowan:

> It's like there's two little people on your shoulders, one saying 'You're doing the right thing, take a deep breath', and the other saying, 'Oh, this is just bollocks'.

Faced with what can feel like an untenable, constantly changing situation, carers move into the polarities of trying to control everything, to keep things as they were, or fall into feeling helpless, overwhelmed by complexity, fearful the river will swirl around them no matter what. However, a strong need to be in control all the time, to avoid a sense of helplessness, can be a short step away from attributing blame to themselves or others.

Working out for themselves, or with others, what they as carers can and cannot control, and must accept ('achieving mastery', relinquishing the fantasy of total control and improving self-care; Boss, 2016) can enable them to stay upright and not be swept away (for now). Focusing on the possible provides small amounts of respite, corners of relaxation; it can restore a sense of quiet competence. It helps develop flexibility and creativity, to enable carers to remember they are people with agency, who can make good choices to improve things for themselves, the parents they care for and others.

Ambiguous loss 9

Caoimhe finds that reducing what she takes on – 'I haven't got the bandwidth for (more), can't deal with any more stress' – is essential, otherwise she gets 'horribly muddled, disorganised feelings'. Making herself do 'exercise I can stand' helps her body, as well as her mind; and 'running low risk, low energy-cost things which raise a bit of money for causes . . . [are] nice because they are out in nature, and that's very calming . . . seeking moments of joy that are about the core of who I am; that doesn't really change'.

Rowan also finds nature a constant source of solace:

Being outdoors always helps, but especially getting in beautifully clear cold water, in a shallow chalk stream pool; it sort of gives me a pinpoint clarity, puts everything into perspective, helps me early in the morning. Wine helps at night! I'd say I was drinking more, it's fine, but it is more.

It's sometimes little things that begin the process of self-care. Carlotta, exhausted from working full-time, trying to sell her house and navigating her mother's constantly changing care package, was existing on adrenaline, and grabbing more and more junk food:

But I know that if I eat rubbish, I feel rubbish. So, I did a HelloFresh order; I wouldn't normally, they're not cheap, but I remembered they were lovely, and it just kick-started me into eating more healthily again. It didn't change anything, but it made me feel a bit better.

All three recognise themselves as individuals with needs, who must look after themselves and re-establish something of their own identify in order to be healthy amidst all the demands and uncertainty. They are experiencing small moments of mastery, and nurturing, which re-ground them in themselves. In this regard, it can be helpful for professionals to support carers to work out what might best enable them to have the 'little life' of their own which Rowan yearns for, alongside their responsibilities as carers dealing with so much, including ambiguous loss.

Who carers connect with in their new situation really matters and may change, some relationships fading as the ambiguous situation unfolds, others becoming more significant. Rowan recognised her losses, and her gains:

I miss Dad's advice; his character changed so much [through dementia]. I can't tell Mum much anymore; she only gets super-anxious. I think I'm less likely to instigate anything social with other friends now, you can't be on the phone all the time if you go out. And . . . I've got a great tag team with my brother, an uncle and an aunt who sends little messages, and is positive and lovely; my partner, who's been through something similar – he'll put a cup of tea beside me when I'm on the phone with Mum, yet again; and my closest friend, she's going through [caring for a parent] too, and we laugh a lot, you have to. But that's about it really.

10   *A. Perry*

Whilst mourning her losses, Rowan and her relatives appear to be working through Boss' principle of 'revising attachments' (2016) in their creation of their 'great tag team'; allowing new connections and a new supportive constellation of roles to emerge between them.

Caoimhe finds space for herself in counselling, breaking out of the isolation often created by ambiguous loss and, in doing so, finds moments of hope and grounding:

> where I can talk with someone who's not emotionally affected by my miserable state . . . then I can unmesh from my mother . . . [it] makes me feel like a separate entity, with space around me; a kind of soul retrieval, not in a shamanistic way, but more psychological, spiritual re-stabilising my sense of self. Remembering who I am . . . coming home to myself.

Carers trying to hold onto the roles they had in relation to the people they are now caring for in exactly the way they used to, is natural but ultimately, futile. Carers have to adapt, experiment, explore doing things differently, respond to the moment (Boss' principle of 'reconstructing identity'; Boss, 2016). Caoimhe noticed that:

> Touch is calming and grounding for her – [her mother] was always a hugger, but I wouldn't pet her, I wouldn't have dared; but that's quite effective now. But de-escalation seems to be most of what I'm doing the whole time . . . it's a curious shift of power . . . hard, because I don't want to lord it over her, but I have to draw the line on some things – our relationship is ambiguous.

Beautifully exemplifying Boss' principle of 'discovering hope'; Boss, 2016), Caoimhe tries to be what she describes as 'sanguine . . . quite a mental process of acceptance, a point of stillness . . . to focus on that, and see it as prizing myself. I live in hope, I think of things I can do'.

There were times, caring for my mother during the lockdown years, that I would find myself muttering and ranting out loud as I went for nightly walks, ruminating on what had and hadn't happened with my father, what was happening with my mother; falling down emotional rabbit holes into many other past losses, shame, blame, disappointments, injustices, self-criticism, self-pity – on and on in a hopeless torrent of mixed feeling and generalisations. Knowing that I had chosen to be their carer had absolutely no impact on this mess of mental, emotional and, at times, physiological distress.

It took a long time and conversations with other adult carers to realise that the very need to rant, and the internal dysregulation doing so out loud represented, was part of the impact of ambiguous loss; the tumbling, whirling thoughts a product of complex and cumulative stress. It took even longer to hear a small voice of self-compassion amidst the clamour, so different from self-pity, and some degree of relaxation. This awareness brings to life Boss' principles (2016) of 'normalising ambivalence' and 'finding meaning', and, as a consequence, 'discovering hope'.

Ambiguous loss 11

Sharing care with my elder brother was my key lifeline. Working with others in community park groups gave me local connection and many things outside the caring situation to hope for and work towards together: physical activity, focus, laughter and fresh air. Supportive conversations and community, and insight into the process we were in together, were enough to enable me to arrive, for the most part, at my mother's door each time in what Caoimhe describes as 'her best self', ready and able, for a while, to be a kind and responsive carer again.

There are so many untold stories of courage quietly happening which should be shared and celebrated together, of those who experience profound ambiguous loss, find meaning and learn to live with it – when they've got the energy. Caoimhe sums up the zigzag path like this:

> It's a kind of . . . spiritual journey and challenge, doing something that tests me . . . I'm willing to accept it, but it's not how I wish my life was at all. I want to be able to regain my control of myself and re-find the love I have and do my best with one of life's many cruelties. Life can be shit as well as life can be great. Most of the time though, honestly, it's not terribly meaningful. My priority is that I don't want to be obliterated by that.

What carers experiencing ambiguous loss need from professionals

Carers meet many professionals coming in and out of their lives alongside the person regarded as the patient; each of those bit part players can have an impact, for good or ill. If each professional had an understanding of ambiguous loss and its potential impact on carers, how they work with them might be of more support. Rowan is having a very mixed experience of professionals:

> The GP is unhelpful, actually . . . patronising, uncaring, no empathy from him. I met with a carers' assessor, just once – she was empathic, seemed to understand what I'm going through, told me I was doing all the right things, which helped, but I've not seen her again. The Vicar, who is brilliant, funny, caring, loves Mum, a good soul. But I'll never forgive the GP for not saying he was sorry about my dad; I don't trust him, but Mum won't change practice.

Working with people who are stressed can be stressful, cumulatively or at times of high tension. Staff working with individuals experiencing ongoing and global ambiguous loss need to ensure their own professional support and self-care strategies are firmly in place (Perry, 2016). I believe that self-awareness is key, as well as knowing when to ask for help (and using it) (Davidson et al., 2022).

A carer's state of dysregulation can dysregulate a professional who needs to stay calm enough to read this as a communication about the carer's internal state, and not react defensively or minimise their concerns. Professionals need to be aware of

12   *A. Perry*

what pushes them out of their window of tolerance (Siegel, 2020) and also know how to bring themselves back inside it.

In the latter months of my father's life, I lost track of the number of professionals who quickly lost their ground around my stressed state; they gave long-winded explanations, talked over me and even snapped. This reinforced my anxiety, creating a spiral of challenge in which neither of us could listen to each other. The exception was the senior nurse from the hospice, who listened with full attention to my incoherent account and said simply: 'Andrea, it's OK. We're here now'. There were still many unpredictable things to work through; but her short comment, spoken quietly and kindly with complete assurance, using my name, reached and calmed me at depth.

In the face of a carer's distress and wish for certainty, professionals may be tempted to agree, or reassure, or acquiesce, give a clearer 'yes' or 'no' in an emotionally charged moment than they might on calmer reflection. They become drawn into the need of carers experiencing ambiguous loss to choose one polarity, for example 'He's no longer capable of doing that alone, is he Doctor?' or the other 'She'll definitely be here for our daughter's wedding, won't she?' (Mannix, 2018).

It is essential for professionals to be aware when their own thinking has been disrupted by stress from any direction (Davidson et al., 2022). When that happens, they need to seek support for themselves to regain a reflective, responsive stance rather than a reactive one. Acknowledging the other's experience is a key part of the psychosocial model described by Davidson et al. (2022) and supports staff to respond appropriately. Thus, before a professional states what is and isn't known about a patient, acknowledging their carer's natural wish for clarity and certainty provides the carer with empathy for their struggle with ambiguous loss, where there is no certainty. For example, phrasing such as the following allows them to deliberately climb down from the professional pedestal and stand alongside carers in ambiguity, whilst trying to identify what might be possible:

> I can see it's hard for you and your brother not to be able to predict how your mum is going to be; entirely natural you'd want me to give you a definite yes or no, I wish I could. And, what I can say at the moment though is that . . .

According to Davidson et al. (2022), this:

- validates the carer's struggle with not knowing, and normalises (I prefer 'naturalises') their distress as a response to ambiguous loss
- enables the carer to feel better regulated, respected, valued, and increases the likelihood they will become able to think more clearly
- reinforces both/and thinking
- points the way to what can be known, and might perhaps be controlled, when so much else cannot, modelling a way to tolerate ambiguity and 'temper mastery'.

Thus, even in short interactions, professionals can draw on Boss' (2016) six principles to support carers struggling with ambiguous loss, towards 'normalising ambivalence', 'tempering mastery', 'finding meaning', and 'discovering hope'.

Perhaps the greatest gift to carers going through ambiguous loss would be for professionals to learn to tolerate ambiguity themselves, in their own lives, so that their empathy is informed by authentic experience.

Conclusion

Carers should rightly expect professionals around them to resource and sustain themselves in such a way that they can offer carers empathically attuned support, cognisant of the impact of ambiguous loss on carers, and on themselves (Nathanson and Rogers, 2020).

Ambiguous loss can isolate carers, very painfully. I hope this chapter, written from both personal and professional perspectives, may help others to find their own pathway to tolerance of ambiguity, meaning and hope, and the professionals alongside them to consider their psychosocial approach to supporting carers.

I am acutely aware that the small cohort of individuals quoted in this chapter are all middle-aged female carers of parents, my own demographic. So, whilst acknowledging that carer experience will likely vary according to the race, ethnicity, identity, gender, relationships, cultural values, beliefs, socioeconomic status, and community context of a carer, I cannot do justice to that breadth of experience. Voices from other carers, including young carers and from diverse groups are of significant value in this field.

References

Boss, P. (2000) *Ambiguous Loss*. Cambridge, MA: Harvard University Press.

Boss, P. (2007) 'Ambiguous loss theory: Challenges for scholars and practitioners', *Family Relations, Special Issue: Ambiguous Loss,* 56(2), pp. 105–110. Available at: https://doi.org/10.1111/j.1741-3729.2007.00444.x.

Boss, P. (2016) 'The context and process of theory development: The story of ambiguous loss', *Journal of Family Therapy Theory and Review,* 8, pp. 269–286. Available at: https://doi.org/10.1111/jftr.12152.

Davidson, S. et al. (2022) 'Supporting staff and volunteers delivering services to people in crisis', in H. Conniff (ed.) *Psychological Staff Support in Healthcare: Thinking and Practice*. Keighley: Sequoia Books, pp. 149–165.

Dupuis, S.L. (2002) 'Understanding ambiguous loss in the context of dementia care', *Journal of Gerontological Social Work,* 37(2), pp. 93–115. Available at: https://doi.org/10.1300/J083v37n02_08.

Hirsch, M.L. (2022) 'What is ambiguous loss and how to cope with it?' Available at: www.everydayhealth.com/emotional-health/what-is-ambiguous-loss-and-how-to-cope-with-it/ (accessed 30 April 2023).

Hughes, D. and Baylin, J. (2012) *Brain-based Parenting: The Neuroscience of Caregiving for Healthy Attachment*. New York: W.W. Norton.

Knight, C. and Glitterman, A. (2019) 'Ambiguous loss and its disenfranchisement: The need for social work interventions', *Families in Society,* 100(2), pp. 164–173. Available at: https://doi.org/10/1177/104438941879937.

Mannix, K. (2018) *With the End in Mind: How to Live and Die Well*. London: William Collins.

Nathanson, A. and Rogers, M. (2020) 'When ambiguous loss becomes ambiguous grief: Clinical work with bereaved caregivers', *Health and Social Work,* 45(4), pp. 268–275. Available at: https://doi.org/10.1093/hsw/hlaa026.

Perry, A. (2016) 'Alongside someone searching: Fulfilling a tertiary attachment role for people looking for lost family', in K-H. Brisch (ed.) *Bindung Und Migration*. Stuttgart: Klett-Cotta.

Siegel, D. (2020) *The Developing Mind*, 3rd edition. New York: Guildford Press.

Tahmazian, R. (2015) *The Agony and the Uncertainty: Missing Loved Ones and Ambiguous Loss*. International Committee of the Red Cross. Available at: www.icrc.org/en/document/agony-and-uncertainty-missing-loved-ones-and-ambiguous-loss (accessed 14 May 2023).

2 Impact on identity for those working as healthcare professionals when taking on the role of carer

Julie Messenger

Introduction

The role and experiences of informal carers are well defined. What is less evident is the impact on identity for those working as healthcare professionals when taking on the role of carer.

Working in healthcare practice does not mean that practitioners are immune from caring responsibilities. Across the UK, many families are now existing as nuclear families rather than as extended family units where responsibility for care is shared across multiple generations of family. Where extended families are absent, the need for partners, parents, or friends to take on care responsibility is massive. For health professionals taking on this role, the role of informal carer is often at conflict with professional roles. This has been highlighted in the literature, for example by Sabyani et al. (2017) who, as part of a systematic review, reflected on seven published sources from which the following five themes were derived:

- Holding privileged knowledge
- Experiencing dilemmas as a consequence of dual identity
- Taking on the role of protector
- Living with family expectations
- Being impacted by the experience.

This chapter is written from the perspective of a practitioner and carer. It will share accounts of how roles and identities changed over time from being that of wife and partner to that of a carer when providing caring support over a sustained period for my husband who experienced life-threatening illness. At its core, this chapter is a demonstration of partnership – at times unequal. It is an account of self-preservation, in particular how easy it is to hide behind a mask created through professional demeanours. The author's hope is that others reading this will be encouraged by the witness and truth shared in this very personal account, feel less isolated and more in control of the challenging situations that they find themselves in.

DOI: 10.4324/9781003435365-2

My story

Writing this was a more challenging activity than I expected. This is a personal account; one that I travelled with my husband as he was, initially, successfully treated for cancer but later went on to present with multiple organ failures (specifically cardiac and renal) due to the chemotherapy he received, which led to his eventual death. It was during the time when he was experiencing multiple organ failures that I took on the role as carer whilst continuing to work professionally as a nurse.

Eight years ago, my husband died. We had been married for 31 years and I truly believe he was my life partner. I thought sufficient time had passed to allow me to write a purposeful account of being a carer as well as a health professional (in my case a qualified nurse and nurse educator with over 40 years of experience), yet the writing was cathartic, churning up so many memories that led me to dispense of many early drafts. I recognise that what I share is personal and unique, reflective of my character, and influenced through my social and professional experiences. I hope that, through sharing my story, others experiencing loss will draw comfort from my reflections and learning.

Box 3. My story

My husband had always been active and well. As his health deteriorated, the eventual diagnosis (after six months of specialist referrals) of a large malignant and cancerous tumour sitting on, or close to, his spine was a shock but, in truth, not unexpected as this potentially helped me understand and explain his symptoms. Being an experienced nurse, once provided with the diagnosis, along with a brief discussion on next steps, I spent hours searching online for treatment options that were showing best results of cure, or leading innovation for this type of cancer. The following morning, I was in the MacMillan treatment centre presenting a consultant oncologist with what I believed they needed to try in terms of treatment! Trust was quickly established when I was informed that this was the treatment that had been ordered the previous evening and would be started later that day. I was fortunate to have an exceptional team leading my husband's care and, after nine months of intensive chemotherapy, intravenously and via lumbar puncture access, he experienced eight years in remission with no return or evidence of cancer. I am forever grateful for this additional time together as earlier discussions around survival were not encouraging given the size and location of the primary tumour.

However, after eight years of good health he collapsed with a heart attack and needed electronic shocking to restore life, immediately requiring stents and a pacemaker to manage cardiac output. Following this, he developed signs of increasing heart and renal failure with doctors attributing earlier chemotherapy as the reason for his deterioration in health. Symptoms were so significant towards end of life that he was only able to walk two or three steps without resting, becoming house-bound and spending increasingly long periods in hospital. When he was at home, I became increasingly reliant on social care so I could continue to work. Throughout this time, I was frustrated and angry through what I saw as poor-quality health and social care; often at times feeling disempowered to seek change.

As a health professional, I was mindful of the opportunities I created to challenge care. I grew increasingly assertive and found I was treated by many as an 'insider' and seen differently from other relatives/carers by those providing health and social care. As I became increasingly confident, I was able to step into the role as advocate to seek health improvements and better quality of care.

Over time I had to recognise that the only outcome for my husband was end of life care, although he harboured expectations of eventual recovery right through to his final week of life. Although I can honestly say that I never want to be as vulnerable and experience loss like this ever again, I have managed to use learning during this time in work and social settings to encourage and support others. I believe I have insight and experience to offer others that would not necessarily have been so pronounced if I had not experienced loss in this way. Rather than protecting this learning, I believe it essential that I should share this to add to the evidence of experience of those providing informal care.

The challenge of being part of a small nuclear family unit

Like many families across the UK, I was in a nuclear family consisting of my husband, son and myself. Our extended families are not local and, therefore, responsibility for care sat entirely with me as I didn't have any buffer of other family members to share in responsibility. In the absence of an extended family, I stepped into the role of carer, without question, leaning on the support of friends. My husband's care needs quickly became complex with our General Practitioner (GP) sharing with us that my husband was the practice's most expensive patient with multiple and deteriorating systems failures – my words and not a direct quotation but this is not something you forget quickly. I felt fortunate that the GP was someone that I knew well, having worked with him while he was a medical registrar and had confidence that he was especially interested and informed on cardiac care. However, hearing that my husband's care was complex and the most serious that they had registered in their practice, led me quickly to understand that this was life-limiting, rather than symptoms that I could expect to see improvements with. At times, it felt that we had a speed dial into medical support and consultation with the consistent need for close monitoring and intervention by health professionals.

18   J. Messenger

Being a carer and health professional – are these roles compatible?

I found that as both a carer and nurse practitioner, I constantly experienced conflict between the roles held and how I viewed my identity. My identity as a wife and mother became blurred, often being overruled by the need to take on the carer's mantle and push for access to care interventions designed to improve health, as well as intervene where I saw, or considered, care as suboptimal.

My experience, although unique, was not dissimilar to that found in the literature. The findings from a systematic review by Sabyani et al. (2017) have informed my reflection. Sabyani et al. examined qualitative articles, published in English, focusing on the experiences of registered nurses or physicians when a significant other was admitted for acute care. This is relatively unchartered territory in that, despite not setting any date restrictions, their review identified only seven papers from which they extracted forty findings. These were collated into five themes as follows:

- Holding privileged knowledge
- Experiencing dilemmas as a consequence of dual identity
- Taking on the role of protector
- Living with family expectations
- Being impacted by the experience.

For the reflection that follows, I found it difficult to separate out the themes as thought processes could have sat under more than one. However, the framework remained a useful tool to comprehensively describe my experience and learning. I suspect if you are reading this having gone through, or experienced similar circumstances, that you may identify with my reflections.

Holding privileged knowledge

There was constant concern over my husband's renal function; however, this was secondary to that of progressive heart failure. Perhaps unsurprisingly, health professionals all assumed that I was knowledgeable on cardiac, respiratory and renal care, despite my clinical area of experience as a nurse being in head and neck surgery. I had to learn quickly in order to feel that I had meaningful conversations, or at least be an accomplished actor to provide the impression that I understood the complexities affecting my husband's care.

I observed that communication with health professionals used professional dialogue and, although I appreciated this level of information, health professionals failed to position the conversation at a level that my husband could easily understand or respond to. He slipped into the role of being a disempowered recipient of care, allowing and expecting me to act as his advocate. I now recognise that I did little to help my husband be an active contributor in meeting his care needs. Without discussing his preferences, I subconsciously took over and often made decisions for him, believing I knew better through being better informed. The importance of

Impact on identity 19

engaging patients in decision-making is well documented. For example, Krist et al. (2017) examined the impact on patients of their involvement in decision-making, behavioural change and chronic disease management and found that involvement improved patients' experience in their health and wellbeing. Through my assertive actions and interventions, as well as the behaviour of other professionals, I shielded my husband from a lot of truth emerging regarding his deteriorating health. I could argue that I was protecting him from what became an increasingly obvious expectation of imminent death, yet I still question how open and transparent I was towards end-of-life care with others and how much of my behaviour was about protecting myself. I will always question whether I got the balance right here but recognise that I cannot change the past, only learn from experiences and move forwards.

From an informed insider's perspective, I have subsequently reflected on the way that others communicated throughout my husband's deteriorating health and eventual death. Possibly due to my assertive personality, I now see how many practitioners directed conversations to me and often spoke over my husband, rather than to him. This was something that I did not pick up on at the time, in part as I looked to absorb as much information as I could to have personal confidence that the care he was receiving, and that which was being considered, was of high quality and evidence based.

The impact of health professionals' language on patient experiences is an area that is well documented. For example, Katz et al. (2022), using a case study approach, examined the impact of language on patient experiences. They suggested that vulnerable individuals could experience poor care resulting from a lack of sensitivity and breaches around confidentiality from ways that information was shared, impacting on trust that is critical to all. Of specific interest, Katz et al. refer to the work of Basile et al. (2021) who reported on what they saw as the dehumanising treatment of patients. Basile et al.'s work focused on patients in Intensive Care who were sedated. They found that health professionals were often observed talking over individuals rather than talking to and with them. Although my husband's circumstances were different, the fact that I was actively involved in many conversations, and as someone in the know, meant that conversations were directed to me due to my professional and assertive manner, marginalising my husband as a potential equal partner. Reflecting back to this time, even though the trajectory of his illness really only had one outcome, that of impending death, I don't believe this message was heard by my husband who, even up to the last week of life, continued to talk about recovery and healing.

Experiencing dilemmas as a consequence of dual identity

I had never seriously considered the concept of identity and the impact that this had on behaviour, perhaps because I had always managed to compartmentalise and separate my identity as a nurse with that of my identity when with family and friends in social situations. With relative ease, I have in the past been able to leave work-related concerns in that environment, thus limiting impact on experiences

20   J. Messenger

outside of work. However, when adopting a carer's role, boundaries between work and home became blurred and increasingly difficult to separate.

There is a growing body of evidence that has examined the consequences of dual identity looking at healthcare professionals stepping into carer roles. For example, one study using phenomenology by Cicchelli and McLeod (2012) looked at the lived experiences of five nurses caring for family members with advanced cancer in Canada. Their findings were not dissimilar to that of my own experiences in that their participants found that the conflict between their professional and personal lives was most challenging; being caught between what they described as 'a web of conflicting expectations' (Cicchelli & McLeod, 2012, p. 53). In this study, the participants spoke about struggles relating to insider knowledge and knowing the illness trajectory, expectations from other health professionals, including those providing the formal care, and expectations within their family units.

I mirrored this sense of conflict and tension, especially the need to balance the role of carer against that of also being an experienced health professional. Did I get this right? I suspect not as I often promoted the professional persona as this made me feel more in control, and safe. However, by doing so, I lost something of my identity as a wife and companion. I became quite detached towards end-of-life in order to safeguard the emotional vulnerability that I was experiencing. Possibly, eight years on, I have still to work through some of this trauma due to loss. I found it possible, and preferable, to hide parts of myself, allowing the professional in me to take over. From my earliest memories of nurse training, I was told that I should not get too emotionally involved with those needing care. I never understood this advice as I naturally look to provide holistic practice, yet I recognise that some level of detachment can be protective and enable professionals to be effective and responsive to the care needs of others. I never expected that I would allow the professional in me to override that of being a wife and companion; yet this was what happened. I felt safe hiding behind a professional persona, protecting myself from dealing openly with difficult emotive issues. This was my way of managing stress and, in many ways, survival. The more I became knowledgeable and insightful with aspects of my husband's deteriorating health, the more apparent his illness trajectory became. When I eventually let down the professional persona and tried to make sense of personal conflicts, imminent emotional trauma, and loss, I found it difficult to remain positive for myself and those close to us. I can see, through revisiting this now, that this had a massive impact on family and friends, with my behaviour at times almost irrational.

Taking on the role of protector

Reflecting back, I saw my role changing from that of being a life partner, to one where I was evidence driven, delving into care and treatment options that I believe should or could be considered. I suspect I was everyone's worst nightmare, pushing for barriers to be lifted so that every option could be considered to optimise my husband's chances for recovery. My pushing of boundaries was often with medical practitioners who, realistically, knew more than me and were better positioned to make appropriate and impartial clinical decisions. As a professional myself, I was

Impact on identity 21

constantly mindful of resourcing challenges with the NHS and the postcode lottery that is often seen, with some patients denied access to treatments due to prohibitive costs. I was clear that one of my key tasks as advocate was to highlight options and get others to make informed decisions as to whether certain treatments would be considered and, if not, why not.

The NHS England Statutory guidance for clinical commissioning groups published in 2017 included the following statement attributed as a personal view of shared decision making: 'I want to feel heard and understood. I want to know about my options, and I want to be supported to make a decision based on what matters to me' (NHS England, 2017, p. 3). Professor Alf Collins, National Policy Advisor in person-centred care, stated that the challenge for health professions was the need to shift the focus of care and support from 'What is the matter with you?' to one that determines 'What matters to you?' (NHS England, 2017, p. 3).

Perhaps due to my extensive experience as a nurse, my husband leant on me with absolute trust that I would seek the best treatment and care options for him. I have the skills to search for leading edge treatments and innovation effectively whereas, I suspect, my husband would have been at a loss to broaden the search beyond well published initiatives. To promote his enhanced wellness, I was not frightened to push ideas around possible treatments that showed signs of promise. Did I raise expectations in others around possible interventions – possibly! Did I take away the locus of self-control from my husband – again possibly, but I did believe I was given implicit permission to do so, needing to get the best treatment considered and hoping that I communicated clearly throughout to optimise partnership working across all parties.

One example of this, as presented in the earlier case summary (Box 3.1), was that I spent several hours researching treatment for Non-Hodgkin's Lymphoma when we were given the initial diagnosis of cancer. This resulted in the discovery of practices that were being championed throughout oncology as leading edge and impacting positively on remission. The next morning, I presented that information to the oncology and haematology consultant only to be assured that this chemotherapy was exactly the treatment that had already been arranged. I don't believe the consultant was surprised by my actions, as he had known of me as a nurse ward manager in the same hospital where my husband was receiving care. I was never one to shy away from what I believed to be right and advantageous to patients. The fact that we were thinking in a similar way helped establish trust. I could let others determine aspects of care knowing that my husband's needs were being recognised and considered. This ultimately helped me through this first phase of illness.

A second example had a very different outcome. During the later stages of heart failure, as his care was heading in the direction of end-of-life provision, although no one had explicitly voiced this yet, my husband was referred for assessment at a specialist cardiac centre to assess suitability for pioneering surgery to improve the function of his mitral valve. Many issues needed to be considered, including travel to the specialist centre and being away from family for a week while under assessment. This would be the first time away from family and friends as all care, until that time, even the specialist chemotherapy years earlier, had been provided locally. Although I was able to visit on a couple of occasions, he had to receive

22   *J. Messenger*

feedback without me as a buffer and was distraught from what he heard. He had entered into this assessment with expectations of a cure or improvement, yet he was eventually informed that the consensus across the specialist team was that if they went through with surgery, and if he survived surgery, that it would be unlikely that they could wean him from the ventilator post-surgery. I couldn't protect him from this and the blunt way it was shared, but I sought to do as much as I could to protect him from similar emotional trauma, even if it meant that, at times, I was not always as transparent as I should have been with information I had gathered or heard.

The two examples above illustrate where I intervened in a protective mode with colleagues who, arguably, were more informed than myself. These next two scenarios sit well within my sphere of influence and relate to quality of care rather than treatment choices.

I hope that this is less evident today but, at the time of my husband's illness, when he needed to spend increasing time in hospital, many of the practice environments were under-resourced and reliant on agency staff to provide necessary nursing care. At the time, I saw myself as almost a 'professional visitor', speculating that I had spent more hours sitting by the bedside in visitors' mode compared to hours spent working clinically. The lack of continuity, due to constant staff changes, meant that it was difficult to form relationships and trust with healthcare professionals as they commonly worked only a single shift. I compensated for this by ensuring that, when I was not working, I spent hours at the hospital, ensuring that he received the care he needed, even if that meant that I was the one providing care to ensure that his needs were met.

Although I am familiar with the clinical environment as a nurse, my position as a carer and advocate meant that I had time to reflect on the quality of care that I saw being practised on and around my husband. It is probably unsurprising if I share that, at a critical point in my husband's illness, I spent more than three hours seeking assurances for improvements in care. The initial triggers for this meeting were when my husband spoke to me distressed as he had been awoken during the night for staff to take blood samples as they had been forgotten on the previous day. Because of his health history, venepuncture was always challenging and rarely did staff find veins easily. In this instance they made six attempts to draw blood unsuccessfully and really traumatised him. The other observation was my own. The hospital operated a protective mealtime policy when a period is set aside for meals with all non-essential activities in practice stopped to protect patients from avoidable interruptions. Unless you helped support feeding, visitors were asked to stay away at this time. These practices are well documented with vulnerable patients often being given food served on red trays to indicate that they require support. Yet what I saw was a disregard for these practices with interventions still taking place; food going cold and, often, necessary feeding support not being provided. With so much known on malnutrition (Stratton, Smith & Gabe, 2018), I was not prepared to sit back and ignore aspects of care that were poor. As stated earlier, I believe I became everyone's personal nightmare, trying to improve care, not just for my husband but for others who didn't have advocates to argue on their behalf.

Living with family expectations

Empirical research has consistently reported on how the carer role can be burdensome and associated with high levels of stress (Schulz & Sherwood, 2008; Biegel, Sales & Schulz, 1991). Haley et al. (1987), perhaps unsurprisingly, showed a direct correlation between levels of stress and individual coping responses and social support experienced by carers. Evidence that the carer's role, for many, can be toxic to health is well reported with many studies examining carers who are supporting mental health, and specifically dementia; however, other longer-term acute and chronic health needs demonstrate similar outcomes in terms of stress and satisfaction (Carers UK, 2022).

I failed to appreciate the impact that the carer role could have on my emotional and physical health. I had always considered that I had effective coping strategies; however, trying to maintain equilibrium being a carer with other responsibilities, particularly being a mother and maintaining a sufficient grasp on work, became all consuming. I coped because that is what I do. I would have been surprised if others had picked up on my vulnerability as I am good at hiding stress. My natural tendency is not to ask others for help or support; therefore, I was challenged when over a short period of only a few weeks, my husband went from being active to being unable, or severely compromised, to meet his own needs. There was no period of transition where we were able to redefine our roles. The transition to the role of carer was sudden, with the speed of health deterioration a surprise even for me as a knowledgeable health professional.

I paid little attention to how the vulnerability and conflict of caring could impact on my career or employment. I remained confident that I had support and sufficient flexibility at work to balance the complexities associated with caring – and there were many! This is not necessarily the experience of others in caring roles. For example, in 2016, Age UK with Carers UK published a document entitled *Walking the Tightrope: The Challenges of Combining Work and Care in Later Life*. This report was commissioned on the, then emerging, evidence that caring has a statistically significant impact on employment for individuals taking on just five hours of caring responsibility weekly, with risks increasing as the responsibility for caring increases further. In the foreword to this document, Helena Herklots, Chief Executive, Carers UK wrote:

> Caring is one of the most important things we do in our lives. We want to do it well. But increasingly we're being asked to combine providing care for family or friends with complex health and care needs at the same time as working to ensure we are financially secure in later life. This collision of responsibilities can put huge pressure on those juggling work and care with negative impacts for their finances, health, and relationships.
>
> (Age UK/Carers UK, 2016, p. 5)

The report found that people aged between 50 and 64 years of age are most likely to be carers and the failure of employers, alongside limited support systems, to help

24   *J. Messenger*

people through transition into caring roles, risks their long-term withdrawal from the labour market, estimated at that time to be costing the UK economy £1.3 billion.

As earlier expressed, I personally didn't feel vulnerable in terms of employment. What did speak to me in this report was an observation of a carer (Age UK/Carers UK, 2016, p. 12) stating that 'I feel like a "push me pull you". . . conflicted, confused . . . But I feel I must not lose track of my own life and role'.

I believe that most people holding caring roles experience these emotions. Whether they do it alone or have others that they can reach out to or are willing to ask for support is critical. For me, it was important that, despite my desire to be there for my husband, stepping in to meet his needs or even, at times, speculating and intervening on what I considered necessary, that I didn't lose myself through this experience. The importance of retaining identity outside the role of carer and being seen as a mother, wife, friend and educated practitioner remained integral.

As expressed above, there were times of conflict, with such an example being in the months leading up to my husband's death. Because of his significant needs, he was entitled to fully funded social care. The package agreed was one that should have allowed me to continue to work, as well as partner with, and support, the social care agencies to provide holistic and individualised care. We had negotiated a package whereby carers would visit twice daily, morning and evening, to support hygiene, nutrition and skin care. By this time, my husband was housebound, confined to the upper rooms of the house, not even having the energy to use a stairlift that had been fitted. Most days, while at work, I would receive a call informing me that no one from the agency had arrived, requiring me to travel home to arrange breakfast and lunch. Often, I would return home to find that he had been left in bed, not supported to the bathroom for washing, or even occasionally, at times when he had attempted to try to be independent, collapsed on the floor. Often at night, support carers failed to attend. I realise that the experience above was unfortunate and possibly not reflective of most of social care but, unlike health care, I felt less sure where to take my concerns and insist on improvements. I worried that if I complained, this would have further detrimental impact on the services offered. This experience, at a time when we were vulnerable, remains with me and is difficult for me to forget. My trust in areas of social care support was severely challenged and, if truth be told, I remain cynical still of their ability to deliver almost a decade on.

Being impacted by the experience

Loss of a life partner after more than three decades together had a major impact on me. A few years earlier I had grieved the loss of a loving parent but this was after many years of illness so, in many respects, I had the opportunity to prepare myself for loss and acceptance of death. This time around, and reflecting on Kübler-Ross' Five Stages of Grieving (Kübler-Ross & Kessler, 2005), each stage was lived out and definitely not in a linear way as often presented in the model, but circular with regular bouts of denial, anger, bargaining, depression and, infrequently, acceptance; commonly experiencing more than one manifestation stage at any one time. I cannot begin to quantify the many weeks when I jointly experienced denial, anger and what I now recognise as depression. It has taken many years, helped by family and friend connections and ongoing life experiences, to get me to the position of what Kübler-Ross refers to as hope.

Learning from grief and loss has been life changing. Having always thrived on being in control, I experienced times when this control was stripped away. I was vulnerable and couldn't hide behind a uniform and professional identity. Although I appreciated that fellow professionals consulted with me as a colleague in the know, there were times when I simply wanted to be a less informed individual and supported, or even led to make appropriate decisions relating to palliative care. Looking back, a good example of this was the morning when a cardiologist invited my husband and I into a consulting room to discuss applying a 'Do not resuscitate' principle to his care. As with many other joint conversations with health professionals, I felt that I was being asked to make the decision when this should have sat with my husband, with support from me. I have thought about this a lot over time and recognise that the locus of control and power over decisions often sat with me rather than with my husband. In retrospect, this was not helpful. I believe, at times, this led to a lack of transparency on prognosis and, until the week of death, a very real and continued belief by my husband that recovery would happen, or was at least possible. For a fiercely independent man, loss of, or having restricted, control must have been difficult.

Resulting from the experience of partnership working and communication, as discussed above, I believe that I am now very sensitive towards ensuring that others are properly listened to and have a voice. This increased sensitivity has been a positive impact in my employment, especially in championing the needs of others and in my role as an experienced academic leader and manager. I now work purposefully to ensure that others in my sphere of influence hold relevant information, allowing them to make decisions for themselves that are informed and appropriate.

Perhaps the biggest impact for me is recognising that it is acceptable to be vulnerable and, in doing so, to ask for support from others, whether this is in a work environment or with family and friends. Letting others in and allowing them to see that I was hurting and not always coping with the pressures of life at that time was difficult. Some of this dates back to learnt behaviours in childhood, but later reinforced when I commenced nurse training. Key messages reinforced during these formative years were about staying strong or portraying an image of strength. In nursing, we were instructed to be dispassionate and stolid when dealing with difficult issues to 'protect ourselves' from hurt, although no one could ever evidence-base this guidance for me.

My behaviour has changed significantly. Through these experiences and hurt, coupled with the love of a great partner, family, and friends, I have ridden this loss and I believe have come out a stronger and more sensitive person than I was in the past. I wouldn't wish my experience on others; however, life throws curveballs at

26 *J. Messenger*

us. I believe strongly that we need to reflect, learn, and can use these to grow and become better persons. Key learning pointers I take from these experiences are:

- Be prepared to be vulnerable.
- Don't assume that you always know best.
- Take others with you every step of the journey, as honestly and transparency are critical.
- Be prepared to have those difficult conversations with those you are caring for.

I believe I am stronger because of these experiences.

References

Age UK and Carers UK (2016) *Walking the Tightrope: The Challenges of Combining Work and Care in Later Life*. Available at: www.ageuk.org.uk/globalassets/age-uk/documents/reports-and-publications/reports-and-briefings/active-communities/rb_july16_walking_the_tightrope.pdf (accessed 10 January 2024).

Basile, M.J. et al. (2021) 'Humanizing the ICU patient: A qualitative exploration of behaviours experienced by patients, caregivers, and ICU staff', *Critical Care Explorations*, 3(6), e0463. Available at: https://doi.org/10.1097/cce.0000000000000463.

Biegel, D.E., Sales, E. and Schulz, R. (1991) *Family Caregiving in Chronic Illness: Alzheimer's Disease, Cancer, Heart Disease, Mental Illness and Stroke*. Newbury Park, CA: Sage Publications.

Carers UK (2022) *State of Caring 2022: A Snapshot of Unpaid Care in the UK*. London: Carers UK. Available at: www.carersuk.org/media/p4kblx5n/cukstateofcaring2022report.pdf (accessed 10 January 2024).

Cicchelli, L. and McLeod, D. (2012) 'Lived experiences of nurses as family caregivers in advanced cancer', *Canadian Oncology Nursing Journal*, 22(1), pp. 53–56. Available at: https://doi.org/10.5737/1181912x2215356.

Haley, W.E. et al. (1987) 'Stress, appraisal, coping, and social support as predicators of adaptational outcome among dementia caregivers', *Psychology and Aging*, 2(4), pp. 323–330. Available at: https://doi.org/10.1037//0882-7974.2.4.323.

Katz, N.T. et al. (2022) 'The impact of health professionals' language on patient experience: A case study', *Journal of Patient Experience*, 9. Available at: https://doi.org/10.1177/23743735221092572.

Krist, A.H. et al. (2017) 'Engaging patients in decision-making and behaviour change to promote prevention', *Studies in Health Technology and Informatics*, 240, pp. 284–302. Available at: www.ncbi.nlm.nih.gov/pmc/articles/PMC6996004/ (Accessed 10 January 2024).

Kübler-Ross, E. and Kessler, D. (2005) *On Grief and Grieving: Finding the Meaning of Grief Through the Five Stages of Loss*. London: Simon and Schuster UK Ltd.

NHS England (2017) *Involving People in their own Health and Care: Statutory Guidance for Clinical Commissioning Groups and NHS England*. Available at: www.england.nhs.uk/wp-content/uploads/2017/04/ppp-involving-people-health-care-guidance.pdf (Accessed 10 January 2024).

Sabyani, H. et al. (2017) 'Experiences of healthcare professionals of having their significant other admitted to an acute care facility: A qualitative systematic review', *JBI Database of Systematic Reviews and Implementation Reports*, 15(5), pp. 1409–1439. Available at: https://doi.org/10.11124/jbisrir-2016-003028.

Schulz, R. and Sherwood, P. (2008) 'Physical and mental health effects of family caregiving', *American Journal of Nursing*, 108(9), pp. 23–27. Available at: https://doi.org/10.1097%2F01.NAJ.0000336406.45248.4c.

Stratton, R., Smith, T. and Gabe, S. (2018) *Managing Malnutrition to Improve Lives and Save Money*. Redditch, Worcestershire, UK: British Association of Parenteral and Enteral Nutrition (BAPEN). Available at: www.bapen.org.uk/pdfs/reports/mag/managing-malnutrition.pdf (accessed 10 January 2024).

3 'I could cry all day, every day, about my losses'

Caring for young adults with life-shortening conditions – families' experiences of disruption and loss

Sarah Earle, Maddie Blackburn, Lizzie Chambers, Julia Downing, Kate Flemming, Jamie Hale, Hannah R. Marston, Lindsay O'Dell, Valerie Sinason and Sally Whitney

Introduction

There are increasing numbers of young people with life-shortening conditions (LSC) who are now surviving into adulthood (Fraser, 2024). This is a heterogenous group with nearly four hundred diagnoses classified as either life-limiting (where there is no reasonable hope of cure) or life-threatening (where curative treatments may be feasible but can fail) in the UK (Noyes et al., 2013). Some of these young adults live near-to-normal lives but more commonly live with episodes of acute illness, chronic pain, and disability; many also have associated cognitive impairment or developmental delay (Together for Short Lives, 2018). Young adults with LSCs often have high care needs, and many of them remain in the family home or rely on family for care. When a child is born with, or develops, a LSC during childhood or adolescence, family carers can experience both material and anticipatory loss. Drawing on a co-produced qualitative study of the experiences of young adults with LSCs and their families during the coronavirus pandemic (Earle et al., 2022; 2024), this chapter focuses on experiences of care and loss among family members. Using an interpretivist approach, and constructivist Grounded Theory Method (cGTM) (Charmaz, 2006; 2014), we draw on thirteen interviews with family members, exploring multiple loss and the intersections between the biographical disruption of caring for someone with a life-shortening illness and the societal disruption of the pandemic response to coronavirus infection.

Background

The canonical concept of biographical disruption was developed by the sociologist Michael Bury (1982) to explore the experiences of adults diagnosed with rheumatoid arthritis. It is based on the fundamental idea that the onset of chronic illness is significant and disruptive; what Giddens (1979) terms a 'critical situation'. Critical

DOI: 10.4324/9781003435365-3

28   S. Earle et.al.

situations can threaten the ontological security of an individual. That is, the 'sense of continuity and order in events' of an individual's life (Giddens, 1984).

The concept of biographical disruption has been widely discussed and critiqued within medical sociology (e.g., Williams, 2000) and applied to multiple experiences of chronic illness, for example, childhood liver disease (Lowton, Hiley and Higgs, 2017), motor neurone disease (Harley and Willis, 2020) and severe sciatica (Saunders, 2018). Biographical disruption refers to the way in which illness is a disruptive experience with 'changes in life situation and relationships' (Bury, 1982, p. 167). Like Bury's original work, most of the research in this field has been applied to those who are chronically ill themselves and few scholars – this chapter being one exception – have focused on biographical disruption by proxy (e.g., see Raymond-Barker, Griffith and Hastings, 2018; Kingod and Grabowski, 2020; Rasmussen, Pedersen and Pagsberg 2020; Boardman and Clark, 2022). This is akin to Goffman's (1963) concept of 'courtesy stigma', stigma experienced by an individual through association with a stigmatised individual. This type of disruption has been described elsewhere as 'parent-biographical disruption' (Rasmussen, Pedersen and Pagsberg, 2020). Here – drawing on the notion of Goffman's concept of courtesy stigma, we use the term courtesy disruption to refer to the disruption experienced by parents through association with their child.

Life-shortening conditions are often characterised by their complexity, unpredictability and uncertain trajectory. The very fact that more children and young people with LSCs are now living into adulthood is illustrative of this and it is for this reason that policy imperatives encourage people with LSCs and their families to engage in 'parallel planning' (NICE, 2016). This refers to how family carers are encouraged to plan for the best (the continuing survival of their child), *and* the worst (their child's inevitable decline and death). Although considered good practice, the concept of parallel planning is not without critics, recognised as 'complex, uncertain [and] emotionally laden' (Morrison, 2020). To date, there is very limited empirical evidence on if, or how, parallel planning takes place in this context. We use the notion of courtesy disruption to inform our thinking about how family members experience caring for a child with a LSC and to consider how material and anticipatory loss feature in their everyday lives, from the point at which symptoms emerge, and a diagnosis is made, through to their child's eventual death.

Coronavirus (COVID-19) emerged sometime in 2019 and by March 2020 a pandemic was declared. In the UK, like in many other parts of the world, governments responded by introducing pandemic control measures such as movement restrictions and lockdowns (Lim, 2021). For those identified as 'clinically extremely vulnerable' – such as many people with LSCs – the government advised them to 'shield' (to stay at home and avoid face-to-face contact with others) in order to protect themselves, and wider society. The media began to widely circulate the information that 'only' older people, and those with pre-existing or underlying health conditions were at risk of dying from COVID-19 (Hastie, 2020). This served to reassure the general population that they were not at risk, while at the same time, positioning old, vulnerable and disabled people as disposable (Abrams and Abbott, 2020). During this time, the NHS also began to ration healthcare, using a Clinical Frailty Scale in a decision-making flowchart to assist clinicians in deciding who would be prioritised for critical care

'*I could cry all day, every day*'   29

(Lewis et al., 2020). Some young people and adults with LSCs were advised by their clinicians that they would not be prioritised for emergency care, including critical care beds or ventilation (Earle et al., 2022). As part of our study, we asked participants to tell us how pandemic control measures such as lockdown, shielding and the rationing of healthcare affected their everyday lives, including the ways in which they planned for the best, and the worst, for their child.

Methods

This chapter draws on a co-produced qualitative research study that set out to investigate the unintended consequences of pandemic control on the lives of young adults living with LSCs and their families in the UK. In total, 40 participants were recruited to the study but, as the focus of this chapter is on carers, only the data pertaining to the experiences of family members are presented here.

Design

Drawing on an interpretive philosophical framework (Kuhn, 1965) the study is informed by constructivist Grounded Theory Methodology (cGTM) (Charmaz, 2006; 2014). It was co-produced by a large multi-disciplinary team that included: three experts by experience (young adults with a LSC; 2 females; 1 gender non-binary), seven female academic researchers (four of whom also had clinical experience) and a policy expert.

Sampling and recruitment

Participants were recruited to the study between June and December 2020 using appropriate inclusion and exclusion criteria (see Table 3.1). In accordance with cGTM, purposive sampling was initially used to recruit participants before using theoretical sampling (Lincoln and Guba, 1985) to saturate emergent categories. We used a range of recruitment methods including advertising in the newsletters of the study partner organisations (*Hospice UK*, *International Children's Palliative Care Network* and *Together for Short Lives*), social media (e.g., Twitter) and the professional, academic, and social networks of the research team – the networks of the experts by experience were particularly helpful. All recruitment was carried out virtually given the need for social distancing and local lockdown rules.

Table 3.1 Inclusion and exclusion criteria

Inclusion criteria	*Exclusion criteria*
Family member of person with a LSC	Not a family member of person with a LSC
Able to communicate in English	Not able to communicate in English
Able to give consent to participate	Not able to consent to participate
Able to participate remotely	Not able to participate remotely
Agree to be audio-recorded	Not agree to be audio-recorded
Living in the UK	Living outside of the UK

30   *S. Earle et.al.*

Participants

We recruited 14 family members to the study; 13 were parents (12 mothers) and one was the partner of a young adult with a LSC. We draw here on the parent data only. Most of the family members were aged between their late 40s to mid-60s. All the participants were White, heterosexual and married except for one, who was divorced. Family members cared for young people and adults aged between the ages of 14 and 34 who had a wide range of LSCs. Most of these young people/adults lived at home (n=9), two lived independently, and two lived in residential care local to the family member.

Data generation and analysis

Data were generated using in-depth interviews (Charmaz, 2014) informed by a topic guide which was amended as the research progressed (Charmaz, 2006; 2014). Online interviews were held between July and December 2020 on Zoom or MS Teams; they were all audio-recorded and transcribed verbatim with consent. Length of interviews varied between 76 and 116 minutes. Six members of the study team – four of the researchers, and two of the experts by experience – took part in interviewing. Interviewers sometimes worked in pairs either because they were not experienced researchers (the experts by experience) or had not previously carried out research with this population group (two of the four academic researchers).

Data were analysed inductively using the constant comparative method (Glaser and Strauss, 1967) and all team members participated in the process of analysis. Data analysis and theoretical sampling were carried out iteratively using line-by-line coding and memoing with the assistance of QSR NVivo 12. Coding was further analysed to generate core categories; some of these categories are represented in this chapter. We stopped interviewing when we had reached theoretical sufficiency (Dey, 2007).

Ethics

Ethical approval was given by The Open University Human Research Ethics Committee in June 2020 (#EARLE/3595). We followed the principle that research consent is a process that is constantly negotiated (Plankey-Videla, 2012) so all participants completed an online consent form and verbal consent was taken again informally during the research process. Participants could decline to answer questions on topics that made them feel uncomfortable and were able to stop or rearrange the interview at any time. All participants were followed up by email within 24 hours post-interview and sent relevant information about support services. Culturally appropriate pseudonyms were chosen to protect participant anonymity. All participants were offered an honorarium (£40 gift voucher) to thank them for their time and contribution to the study.

Findings

Four key categories were identified through analysis highlighting the courtesy disruption brought about by the material and anticipatory losses experienced by parents who care for a child with a LSC. These are: a loss of certainty and ontological security; the loss of idealised notions of babies and parenthood; the loss of future(s); and the anticipatory loss of an idealised good death.

Loss of certainty and ontological security

Life-shortening conditions can become apparent either before or when a baby is born – for example, through genetic testing, a problematic pregnancy, or complicated delivery. Other conditions become evident shortly after birth or in infancy and some develop later in childhood or in adolescence. Family members begin to experience the loss of certainty and ontological security at different times depending on when their child showed symptoms of, or was diagnosed with, a LSC.

Mary's son, Oliver, has a medically complex and rare genetic syndrome. Shortly after he was born, she was told that he probably would not live beyond his first year of life:

> the first year of their lives a 95% death rate, but as he's got older obviously he's got better . . . we were told Oliver was a no hoper, and that they probably didn't think he would survive.
>
> (Mary, in her 50s, mother to Oliver, mid-teens)

In contrast, in David's case, his daughter Tabitha, who is now in her early 30s, lived a relatively normal life until her late teens and it was then that symptoms emerged:

> I mean this started probably when she was 17. . . and from then on the difficulties set in as we tried to understand what happened to this erstwhile very fit and still very bright girl as to what the bloody hell's gone on. I guess the first eight or nine years, it was just trying to sort the procedural stuff out because we didn't know what was wrong with her and then we did know what was wrong, we didn't know what to do with that diagnosis.
>
> (David, in his 60s, dad to Tabitha, mid 30s)

David describes how they '*lurched from specialist to specialist*' until – many years later – a diagnosis was given. In some instances, a diagnosis can have repercussions for other children within a family. For example, when Tina's daughter, Patsy (now aged 30), was diagnosed with a LSC in her 20s, this meant it 'then gave the diagnosis to her sister as well'.

Following diagnosis, the prognosis of many LSCs is typically evolving and ambiguous and, in some cases, symptoms are not definitively diagnosed, leading to ongoing uncertainty, sometimes for the duration of a child's life. Family members often use familiar tropes and illness metaphors to manage and describe the ongoing but uncertain survival of their children:

> His prognosis was very poor, in as much as they thought that if he did well, children like this who do well survive to puberty, and he's 29. So like a lot of our young people, he's beaten all the odds.
>
> (Barbara, in her 60s, mother to Kevin, late 20s)

32   *S. Earle et.al.*

Initially they thought that her life expectancy would be around 12 and then they said maybe 16 or 17. So for us to get to 22 is just a miracle really.. . . So, she's a real toughie and a real fighter.

(Lynne, in her 60s, mum to Belinda, early 20s)

So, she's had quite a few close shaves, I think she's a cat with nine lives, but she's rapidly running out of them.

(Erin, in her 50s, mother to Clara, early 30s)

The loss of certainty and ontological security begins with the diagnosis of symptoms that are recognised as life-shortening, even when achieving a diagnosis takes many years, if at all. The uncertain prognosis that is typical of many LSCs extends this uncertainty throughout a child's life, and can have unsettling implications for others, such as siblings.

Loss of idealised notions of babies and parenthood

When a child is diagnosed with a LSC, family members begin to experience the loss of idealised notions of babies and parenthood. This type of loss speaks to the way in which expectant parents imagine their future child, their relationship with that child and the life they will share both together and separately.

Lynne spoke about the loss of her imagined future with a new baby and the grieving process when her baby was technically stillborn and then survived. She describes her daughter, as 'medically complex, profoundly severely disabled, with severe learning disabilities and a diagnosis as long as your arm':

You know, when you're pregnant you have all these wonderful plans about what you're going to do with your baby.. . . So when we had Belinda obviously those plans were completely shattered.. . . I could sit and I could cry all day every day about my loss. Because I guess in some ways Belinda was born and she wasn't what I thought she was going to be so it's a grieving process isn't it. But she's an absolute blessing.

(Lynne, in her 60s, mum to Belinda, early 20s)

Like many family members, Lynne describes a deep loss on learning that her child would be profoundly disabled but – at the same time – is keen to emphasise the positives, describing her daughter as a 'blessing'. Other participants made similar comments, for example one described her son as 'one of the happiest people I've ever met' and another reflected on how her 'life would be weird without' her son.

Many family members spoke about the impact of their child's illness on their own lives, particularly the impact this had on work and careers. Some participants gave up work temporarily to care for their child, before later retraining and returning to the workforce. Others simply gave up work to care for their child on a permanent and full-time basis, for example, Doris says:

I had to be medically retired when my daughter was five when she had cancer the second time because I needed to look after her. So, I got medically retired from my job and I've cared for her ever since.

(Doris, in her 60s, mother to Henrietta, late 20s)

All family members provided care for their child, even when that child was living outside of the family home. This caring role made it difficult for some participants to identify with a parenting (mothering) role. For Lily, it is her relationship with her other (non-disabled son), John, which enables her to fulfil her mothering role, describing themselves as 'best of mates':

I've got a 28-year-old, John. To me he feels like an only child.. . . You know, I don't feel like mum half the time with Elena, I feel like carer. Whereas with John I'm mum all the time. No matter what happens I'm still mum . . . . It's mum and son. Best of mates.

(Lily, in her 40s, mother to Elena, early 20s)

In contrast, some family members struggled to identify as carers. Erin, for example, whose daughter lived independently, saw herself simply as a mother:

I'm just her mum . . . so we've got this carer's group in work and no I don't, because I'm just doing what your mum does. Yeah, it's stupid I know, I know that's actually what I am [a carer], but yeah. It's complex . . . how do you unpick that relationship between mum and being a carer?

(Erin, in her 50s, mother to Clara, early 30s)

One family member – David – rejected the carer role, expressing ambivalence about what it means to be 'a carer'. It is interesting to note that David is the only father within the study:

I said to my wife when we realised that she was going to need care long term that I was not a carer, but I was her father. And she sort of baulked at that.

(David, in his 60s, dad to Tabitha, mid-30s)

Trajectories of biographical disruption differ depending on when it becomes apparent that a child has a LSC. In some cases, it is immediately apparent that a child will have complex needs and in others, symptoms begin to emerge later. This unexpected change to an idealised norm of babies and parenting serves to disrupt plans and hopes for the future including the disruption of parental identities.

Loss of future(s)

Following the diagnosis of a LSC, family members typically describe the trajectory of their child's life as 'unknown'. This uncertainty, together with the expectation of parallel planning – planning for the best, while preparing for the worst – is disquieting and makes it difficult to look to the future.

34   *S. Earle et.al.*

We asked family members to tell us about their experience of parallel planning. Some family members recognised that the early death of their child was inevitable, even if it was something that they chose not to dwell on often. Like most participants, David found the subject difficult to talk about:

> The fact is that she has a much higher chance of early death, maybe dying before I do.. . . And that's difficult, but that's life, or indeed, that's death. And you can't go down the rabbit hole of 'why has it happened to my daughter?'. . . That's not the way to handle it, you can't do it.
>
> (David, in his 60s, father to Tabitha, mid-30s)

Several participants said that they had not discussed parallel planning at home. A reluctance to talk about end-of-life was typically framed within the context of their child being 'really well', or 'doing OK', thus minimising the need to talk about death. For example:

> [This is] not something we discuss. Even in our house, we don't discuss that. God forbid that ever happened. But Oliver seems to be doing OK.
>
> (Mary, in her 50s, mother to Oliver, mid-teens)

Some families talked about having advance care plans, although they saw it as something that had been 'done' (and put away) rather than as an ongoing process. In several instances, advance care planning had been undertaken as part of the transition from children to adult services and, since that time, had not been revisited. Michelle said:

> No, nobody's ever mentioned it [advance care planning] since we stopped using the hospice.. . . I don't know, I think it's, sometimes we almost have to remind ourselves that Ian's got this condition, because during the day when he's up and about he does lead an almost normal life.. . . I'm not sure if that's irresponsible or not, I don't know.
>
> (Michelle, in her 50s, mother to Ian, early 30s)

At times – particularly at a time of crisis – revisiting parallel planning comes to the fore. At the time of interview, Rachael's son, Anthony, was having an emergency brain scan, following chemotherapy treatment for a renal tumour:

> I struggle with the advanced care directive, end-of-life stuff obviously, but we have to think about that. It could be a discussion I'm having tomorrow afternoon with his neurologist again . . . . I just try not to visit it too regularly for my own sanity, but it's always there.
>
> (Rachael, late 40s, mother to Anthony, early 20s)

Overall, most participants avoided dwelling on the likely early death of their child and preferred to focus on more immediate concerns. For example:

'I could cry all day, every day' 35

Well, honestly, we don't look that far ahead. I would say I look five years ahead with Finnley.... Looking at the future that far ahead does scare me.
(Tabitha, in her 50s, mother to Finnley, late teens)

The pandemic accentuated the tendency to focus on living in the moment, rather than thinking about an uncertain and undesirable future. For example:

I think it's underlined my thinking that you have to live for the moment. You can't plan too far ahead.... So yeah, I think that's, it's a message for us all isn't it?
(Rachael, late 40s, mother to Anthony, early 20s)

The ongoing uncertainty of caring for a child with a LSC meant that looking to the future was difficult and, often, avoided. The findings suggest that some family members had engaged with parallel planning, but many found it difficult to talk about. The pandemic heightened a sense of living in, and for, the moment against the threat of potential COVID infection.

Loss of an idealised 'good death'

Although family members found it difficult to talk about the death of their child and most avoided discussion of parallel planning, it was clear that the majority had given some thought to how and where they would like their child to die. During interviews we asked participants to talk about the effect (if any) of the pandemic on their end-of-life planning. It was clear that the pandemic was disrupting this, although not everyone wanted to consider it. For example, one participant said:

I haven't even thought about it because I couldn't bear to think about it. It would be horrendous.
(Doris, in her 60s, mum to Henrietta, late 20s)

Although participants recognised that the death of their child was, eventually, inevitable, dying from COVID was seen as preventable and avoidable. Lily says:

I think my biggest fear has always been, with Elena, losing her to something that I can prevent. If I can prevent it, there's no need for it to happen.
(Lily, in her 40s, mum to Elena, early 20s)

Like Lily, Lynne was focused on keeping her daughter safe and did not want to consider the need for alternative end-of-life plans:

I'm here to keep Belinda safe. So, I just have got in a complete mindset of this is our life, this is what it is at the moment.... This is the way that I'm keeping Belinda alive . . . So, this, as far as I'm concerned I have no alternative.... I've just dug deep and get on with it.
(Lynne, in her 60s, mum to Belinda, early 20s)

36   S. Earle et.al.

Family members were aware that COVID restrictions might impact on end-of-life plans and that options previously available to them might not be. They were also aware of the prioritisation of healthcare within hospitals, particularly access to ventilation and critical care. For example:

> I think to start with we were all very worried for him, because what the doctor said made perfect sense. That they wouldn't ventilate Anthony and they didn't think his lungs and kidneys would cope.
>
> (Rachael, in her 40s, mother to Anthony, early 20s)

> It was difficult in the beginning, because NICE were thrashing out these guidelines, weren't they? There was the frailty scale, you know, if there was a shortage of oxygen . . . if the hospital is overloaded, then Ewan being in the state he was, they wouldn't have taken him in.
>
> (Bronwyn, in her 50s, mum to Ewan, late teens)

Participants were particularly fearful of the idea that – because of COVID restrictions – their child might die alone. Jessica's response was typical of this:

> I think my main thing is that if she did get ill and she was in hospital, I would be absolutely insistent that she was never on her own. I'd stay with her 24 hours if I had to.
>
> (Fiona, late 40s, mother to Jessica, late teens)

Barbara's son Kevin lived in residential care. Like other family members, she wanted her son to die in a familiar setting and was surprised that the care home would choose to send her son to hospital where he would be isolated and alone:

> If he was to become ill with COVID and our discussions at the time was not to be admitted, not to be ventilated, not to be separated from the family but to be given palliative care.. . . And then I talked to the manager of the care home . . . who was all a bit shocked and said 'well, obviously if he gets ill he'll go straight into hospital'. I said 'I don't think that's how it's going to work'. . . we don't want him to be there isolated, scared, completely cut off on his own.
>
> (Barbara, in her 60s, mother to Kevin, late 20s)

In the following extract Lily expresses real ambivalence about what she wants for her daughter, Elena, should she become unwell. On the one hand, she wants her daughter to survive but does not want her to die alone.

> it's written everywhere for everybody wherever she goes, if she suddenly stopped breathing you keep her alive until I get there. Because I do not want her to pass without me being there, I need to be with her . . . she'll be staying here. She will die here where she knows everyone. Yeah, she won't be dying anywhere else.
>
> (Lily, in her 40s, mum to Elena, early 20s)

'I could cry all day, every day' 37

Although family members found it very hard to talk about the subjects of death and dying, they had developed the concept of a good death for their child. For many, the disruption brought about by the pandemic threatened this concept and led to fear and uncertainty about what might happen. For others, the focus was on keeping their child safe through the pandemic and could not bring themselves to think about losing their child to something they regarded as preventable.

Discussion and conclusion

This chapter has explored the material and anticipatory losses experienced by family members who care for a child with a LSC and the way in which some of these losses are amplified by the pandemic. At the time the interviews took place, the pandemic control measures predominantly appeared to impact on concerns around planning for end of life and what might be feasible in relation to a good death given the controls in place in hospitals and hospices.

When a child becomes ill and is then diagnosed with a LSC, family members experience a disruption to their ontological security (Giddens, 1984). That is, they no longer have the stability and certainty they once had prior to the disruption brought into their lives by their child's illness. Bluebond-Langner (1996) describes this as living in the 'shadow of illness', something that can also affect others, such as siblings. However, our study highlights how family members, in the context of the loss of certainty and ontological security, also seek to normalise their experiences and find the positives amidst the disruption of life-changing illness.

Life-shortening conditions are often in flux, characterised by periods of stability, followed by episodes of acute illness, including life-threatening events. The loss of certainty and security can be gradual or immediate, depending on when and how symptoms emerge, and (whether) a diagnosis is made. This uncertainty leads to a form of courtesy disruption, or parent-biographical disruption (Rasmussen, Pedersen and Pagsberg, 2020), which threatens the identity of family members and the imagined future(s) for themselves and their child. The loss of idealised notions of babies and parenthood can, however, come to be replaced by a carer identity, although this is not uncomplicated.

Our study shows how family members often describe the trajectory of their child's life as '*unknown*' and most were mindful of the need to plan for the best, *and* the worst, for their child. The 'parallax' (Žižek, 2006), a concept used by MacArtney et al., (2017) to describe both the liminality and positive actions required to navigate living and dying at the end of life, is useful here. Most family members found the idea of parallel planning very challenging. Some research participants did not want to talk about it, and became pensive and tearful during interviews, although all of them were willing to discuss the topic with us when prompted. Although family members were resistant to the idea of advanced care, or end-of-life planning, the pandemic underlined the importance of this but made them fearful for the life, and death, of their child.

There is a considerable body of literature on the notion of a 'good death' (see Kellehear, 1990) and it is a central tenet of the hospice movement (Hart, Sainsbury and Short, 1998). The good death has been subject to considerable criticism

38   S. Earle et.al.

but holds a diversity of meanings and interpretations. Pandemic restrictions and the threat of COVID-19 threatened participant's plans for a good death and ensuring that their child did not die alone was prevalent across accounts. Although early death is non-normative, parents of children with a LSC develop a new normal; that their child will die, eventually, from their condition and this forms part of a revised normality, integrated into their biographies. The possibility of dying from COVID disrupted this new normal; it was seen as unacceptable and regarded as a preventable, bad death.

All research studies have strengths and limitations. We felt fortunate to interview participants about their experiences of everyday life during the pandemic, at a time of considerable personal and social crisis and uncertainty. To our best knowledge, it is the only co-produced qualitative study of its kind in the UK during the pandemic. However, our study group was predominantly female, heterosexual and White meaning that some groups are not well represented within the data.

This study is not exhaustive in its analysis of the courtesy disruption and material and anticipatory losses experienced by family members who care for those with a LSC. Greater attention to gender, disruption and loss would be advantageous as would a focus on non-White populations, especially since epidemiological studies suggest that the prevalence of such conditions is highest among young people of Pakistani, other Asian and Black origins (Gibson-Smith et al., 2021).

Acknowledgements

Thank you to our research participants and to the late Lucy Watts, who also contributed to this project.

References

Abrams, T. and Abbott, D. (2020) 'Disability, deadly discourse, and collectivity amid Coronavirus (COVID-19)', *Scandinavian Journal of Disability Research*, 22(1), pp. 168–174. Available at: http://dx.doi.org/10.16993/sjdr.732.

Bluebond-Langner, M. (1996) *In the Shadow of Illness: Parents and Siblings of the Chronically Ill Child*. Princeton, NJ: Princeton University Press.

Boardman, F. and Clark, C. (2022) '"We're kind of genetic nomads": Parents' experiences of biographical disruption and uncertainty following in/conclusive results from newborn cystic fibrosis screening', *Social Science and Medicine*, 301, 114972. Available at: https://doi.org/10.1016/j.socscimed.2022.114972.

Bury, M. (1982) 'Chronic illness as biographical disruption', *Sociology of Health and Illness*, 4(2), pp. 167–182. Available at: https://doi.org/10.1111/1467-9566.ep11339939.

Charmaz, K. (2006) *Constructing Grounded Theory: A Practical Guide through Qualitative Analysis*. London: Sage.

Charmaz, K. (2014) *Constructing Grounded Theory*, 2nd edition. London: Sage.

Dey, I. (2007) 'Grounding categories', in A. Bryant and K. Charmaz (eds) *The Sage Handbook of Grounded Theory*. Los Angeles: Sage, pp. 167–190.

Earle, S. et al. (2022) '"Whose life are they going to save? It's probably not going to be mine!" Living with a life-shortening condition during the Coronavirus (COVID-19) Pandemic: A grounded theory study of embodied precarity', *Qualitative Health Research*, 32(14), pp. 2055–2065. Available at: https://doi.org/10.1177/10497323221131692.

Earle, S. et al. (2024) 'Disruptions, relationships and intimate futures: The unintended consequences of pandemic control', in S. Earle and M. Blackburn (eds) *Sex, Intimacy and Living with Life-Shortening Conditions*. Abingdon: Routledge.

Fraser, L. (2024) 'A changing population: Young adults with life-limiting or life-threatening conditions', in S. Earle and M. Blackburn (eds) *Sex, Intimacy and Living with Life-Shortening Conditions*. Abingdon: Routledge.

Gibson-Smith, D. et al. (2021) *Making Every Young Adult Count*. York: University of York.

Giddens, A. (1979) *Central Problems in Social Theory*. London: Macmillan.

Giddens, A. (1984) *The Constitution of Society: Outline of the Theory of Structuration*. Oakland, CA: University of California Press.

Glaser, B.G. and Strauss, A.L. (1967) *The Discovery of Grounded Theory: STRATEGIES for Qualitative Research*. New York: Aldine de Gruyter.

Goffman, I. (1963) *Stigma: Notes on the Management of Spoiled Identity*. Eaglewood Cliffs, NJ: Prentice-Hall.

Harley, K. and Willis, K. (2020) 'Living with motor neurone disease: An insider's sociological perspective', *Health Sociology Review*, 29(2), pp. 211–225. Available at: https://doi.or g/10.1080/14461242.2020.1789487.

Hart, B., Sainsbury, P. and Short, S. (1998) 'Whose dying? A sociological critique of the "good death" ', *Mortality*, 31(1), pp. 65–77. Available at: https://doi.org/10.1080/713685884.

Hastie, J. (2020). *Covid-19: A Plea for our Lives*. Available at: https://youtu.be/EcRtAsdpg30 (accessed: 10 August 2023).

Kellehear, A. (1990) *Dying of Cancer: The Final Year of Life*. Melbourne: Harwood Academic Publishers.

Kingod, N. and Grabowski, D. (2020) 'In a vigilant state of chronic disruption: How parents with a young child with type 1 diabetes negotiate events and moments of uncertainty', *Sociology of Health and Illness*, 42(6), pp. 1473–1487. Available at: https://doi. org/10.1111/1467-9566.13123.

Kuhn, T.S. (1965) 'Logic of discovery or psychology of research?', in I. Lakatos and A. Musgrave (eds) *Criticism and the Growth of Knowledge: Proceedings of the International Colloquium in the Philosophy of Science*. London: Cambridge University Press, pp. 1–24.

Lewis, E.G. et al. (2020) 'Rationing care by frailty during the COVID-19 pandemic', *Age and Ageing*, 50(1), pp. 7–10. Available at: https://doi.org/10.1093/ageing/afaa171.

Lim, W.M. (2021) 'Editorial: History, lessons, and ways forward from the COVID-19 pandemic', *International Journal of Quality and Innovation*, 5(2), pp. 101–108. Available at: www.inder-science.com/info/dl.php?filename=2021/ijqi-7348.pdf (accessed 6 February 2024).

Lincoln, Y.S. and Guba, E.G. (1985) *Naturalistic Enquiry*. London: Sage.

Lowton, K., Hiley, C. and Higgs, P. (2017) 'Constructing embodied identity in a 'new' ageing population: A qualitative study of the pioneer cohort of childhood liver transplant recipients in the UK', *Social Science and Medicine*, 172, pp. 1–9. Available at: https://doi. org/10.1016/j.socscimed.2016.11.015.

MacArtney, J.I. et al. (2017) 'The liminal and the parallax: Living *and* dying at the end of life', *Qualitative Health Research*, 27(5), pp. 623–633. Available at: https://doi. org/10.1177/1049732315618938.

Morrison, R.S. (2020) 'Advance directives/care planning: Clear, simple, wrong', *Journal of Palliative Medicine,* 23(7), pp. 878–879. Available at: https://doi.org/10.1089/ jpm.2020.0272.

NICE (2016) *End of Life Care for Infants, Children and Young People with Life-Limiting Conditions: Planning and Management* (NICE guideline NG61). Available at: www.nice. org.uk/guidance/ng61 (accessed: 10 August 2023).

Noyes, J. et al. (2013) 'Evidence-based planning and costing palliative care services for children: Novel multi-method epidemiological and economic exemplar', *BMC Palliative Care,* 12(1), 18. Available at: https://doi.org/10.1186/1472-684X-12-18.

Plankey-Videla, N. (2012) 'Informed consent as process: Problematizing informed consent in organizational ethnographies', *Qualitative Sociology*, 35, pp. 1–21. Available at: https://doi.org/10.1007/s11133-011-9212-2.

Rasmussen, P.S., Pedersen, I.K. and Pagsberg, A.K. (2020) 'Biographical disruption or cohesion? How parents deal with their child's autism diagnosis', *Social Science and Medicine*, 244, 112673. Available at: https://doi.org/10.1016/j.socscimed.2019.112673.

Raymond-Barker, P., Griffith, G.M. and Hastings, R.P. (2018) 'Biographical disruption: Experiences of mothers of adults assessed for autism spectrum disorder', *Journal of Intellectual and Developmental Disability*, 43(1), pp. 83–92. Available at: https://doi.org/10.3109/13668250.2016.1262011.

Saunders, B. et al. (2018) 'Biographical suspension and liminality of self in accounts of severe sciatica', *Social Science and Medicine*, 218, pp. 28–36. Available at: https://doi.org/10.1016/j.socscimed.2018.10.001.

Together for Short Lives (2018) *A Guide to Children's Palliative Care*, 4th edition. Bristol, UK: Together for Short Lives. Available at: TfSL-A-Guide-to-Children's-Palliative-Care-Fourth-Edition-FINAL-SINGLE-PAGES.pdf (accessed 29 January 2024).

Williams, S. (2000) 'Chronic illness as biographical disruption or biographical disruption as chronic illness? Reflections on a core concept', *Sociology of Health and Illness*, 22(1), pp. 40–67. Available at: https://doi.org/10.1111/1467-9566.00191.

Žižek, S. (2006) *The Parallax View*. Cambridge, MA: MIT Press.

4 From physically active to physically inactive

Understanding the experiences of a familial carer's loss of self

Nichola Kentzer, Martin Penson and Melinda Spencer

Introduction

Research has considered the transition to caring through several lenses including Bury's biographical disruption (Lopes De Melo et al., 2020), van Gennep's liminality theory (Gibbons et al., 2014) and Montgomery and Kosloski's (2009) caregiving identity theory (Beatie et al., 2019). This chapter aims to extend existing literature and contribute further knowledge of the caregiving experience by examining the transition into caring, leading to a loss of self, of Martin, participant, co-researcher and second author. More specifically, the chapter explores Martin's loss of athletic identity with the change to his 'new' identity as a carer to his mum, a stroke survivor. This unique perspective allows us to draw on a body of literature from the field of sport in terms of athlete transitions. This case discussion also presents a different insight into the barriers and facilitators to being physically active in the caring role, an under-researched area in the UK (Horne et al., 2021), from a carer who previously had physical activity (PA) firmly at the centre of his life.

In the United Kingdom (UK), the value of unpaid care is equivalent to a second National Health Service (NHS) in England and Wales (approximately £164 billion) with people providing more hours of unpaid care than ever before (Petrillo and Bennett, 2022), often to family members. Indeed, it is expected that family carers will continue to be the main source of care for many people in both developed and developing countries because of increases in life expectancy, chronic illnesses, and associated dependency (OECD, 2019).

While there is evidence of positive outcomes from caring such as strengthening relationships, a sense of fulfilment and satisfaction, emotional rewards, and personal growth (Lloyd, Patterson and Muers, 2016), caring can negatively impact on carers' health, social life, employment, and finances (Larkin, Henwood and Milne, 2019). According to Harris (2020, p. 3), these are areas that are "most likely to assault our deeply held views of the world and ourselves".

Two-thirds of carers report that they have focused on the care needs of the person they care for, rather than their own needs (Carers UK, 2019). It is perhaps unsurprising, therefore, that carers can experience negative emotional experiences (Malewezi et al., 2022) including loneliness (Willis, Vickery and Symonds, 2020), anxiety (Kaddour and Kishita, 2020) and depression (del-Pino-Casado et al., 2021).

DOI: 10.4324/9781003435365-4

Poorer physical health is also reported, including back pain and high blood pressure (Larkin, Henwood and Milne, 2019). Moreover, poorer physical and mental health outcomes are influenced by the number of hours of care provided (Brimblecombe et al., 2018) as well as gender, ethnicity, socio-economic status, and age of the carer (Brimblecombe and Cartagena Farias, 2022).

Another factor that impacts on the caring role is the condition of the care recipient and whether there is a gradual or sudden transition into the caring role. For example, the sudden onset of a stroke in addition to its unpredictable and complex recovery, can make it difficult for family members to adjust in their caring role (Saban and Hogan, 2012). Indeed, carers taking on this unexpected role describe a sense of loss relating to self-identity, and of relationships with the person they care for and friends and family (Eifert et al., 2015).

Carers and physical activity

Physical activity (PA) is defined "as any bodily movement produced by skeletal muscles that requires energy expenditure" (World Health Organisation; WHO, 2010) and contributes to improved physical and mental health, the reduction of risk of multiple chronic diseases, as well as providing benefits for mood, sleep, and quality of life (WHO, 2020). Despite these published benefits, WHO (2022) report that more than 80% of adolescents and more than one in four adults do not meet their recommended levels of physical activity for optimum health.

Concerningly, research suggests that carers engage in less PA when they become a carer (Cao et al., 2010; Ross et al., 2020), and it is important to highlight that carers report that they are less active than they would like (Carers UK, 2019; 2021). A systematic review by Lindsay et al. (2022) found conflicting results when comparing carers and non-carers' PA levels. The authors discussed the difference between types of PA, for example considering the benefits to health of leisure PA, but the potential detriment to health of PA within the caring role.

It has been suggested that the "psychosocial experience of PA, rather than the energy expenditure" is important to carers (Loi et al., 2016, p. 299). Indeed, Piggin's (2020, p. 5) definition of PA acknowledges that being physically active goes beyond the body and includes a more holistic and contextual explanation:

> Physical activity involves people moving, acting, and performing within culturally specific spaces and contexts, and influenced by a unique array of interests, emotions, ideas, instructions and relationships.

This more complex picture of PA is reflected by the findings of Carers UK (2022) that carers with poorer physical and mental health, those struggling financially, those from an ethnic minority background, those caring for more than 50 hours per week and those who experience loneliness, are less active. In their research examining PA in carers aged 55 and over in England, Carers UK (2021) reported that men were slightly more likely to be active than women – reflecting the wider population.

From physically active to physically inactive 43

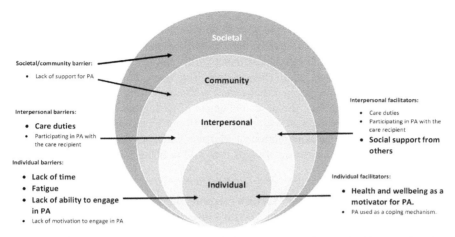

Figure 4.1. Socioecological model of the barriers and facilitators to carers' PA
Source: (Lindsay et al., 2023, p. 516).

Participation barriers to PA, such as guilt, have been reported more widely in the literature, along with lack of time, fatigue, and care duties (Horne et al., 2021). To better understand existing influences on PA, and how these interact, Lindsay et al. (2023) categorised and mapped the barriers and facilitators from the perspective of carers to the socioecological model identified in their systematic review (see Figure 4.1).

With carers being in worse health than the overall population, there is a clear need to support carers to be more active so they can benefit from the positive health effects of physical activity (Carers UK, 2023; Martis et al., 2023).

Transitioning to a physically inactive caring role

With evidence suggesting that carers become less active upon taking on a caring role, an examination of sport transition research could help facilitate a better understanding of the changing relationship with PA that carers can experience. There are several transitions that athletes experience during their career before they end their career in retirement (Stambulova, Ryba and Henriksen, 2021). It could be argued, therefore, that a carer could experience a transition 'out' of their previously more physically active lifestyle – a concept that has not been examined to date.

Sport transition research informs us that athletes who maintained a sport/life balance and are ready for retirement are more likely to experience a positive final transition out of their sport (Fairlie et al., 2019). Further, social support is fundamental for a positive transition (Brown et al., 2018). Those athletes with a stronger athletic identity and those experiencing forced transitions can face greater

44   *N. Kentzer et al.*

challenges, including periods of psychological distress (Demetriou et al., 2020). Indeed, if an athlete's involvement in their sport is threatened, there can be a tendency for them to dissociate from their identification to avert the cost of having to adjust (Brewer et al., 2010). Unfortunately, this can lead to a feeling of a sense of loss and poorer mental health (Sanders and Stevinson, 2017).

From this it could be posited that carers with an existing identity grounded in being active, not only face the new challenges of caring but also the impact of a loss of identity, one associated with physical activity. This chapter seeks to explore this concept through an examination of Martin's caring experiences, as he transitioned from being physically active (see Box 4.1) to being physically inactive.

Box 4.1:   Understanding Martin's relationship with PA before his transition to being a carer (extracts from Martin's interview/diary in quotation marks)

Martin's mum suffered a severe stroke in 2016 and he, an only child aged 53, immediately stepped back from his work, to become her full-time carer. He was located rurally, over 20 miles to the closest carer centre, and cared for his mum until her passing in January 2020.

'Physical health and fitness had always played a significant part' in Martin's lifestyle choices and was an aspect of his life that he 'particularly enjoyed and gained a great deal of satisfaction from'. In addition to the physical benefits, PA provided a 'means of socialising and a close network of training colleagues/ friends was established over the years'. Such was the significance of PA, exercise, and sport in his life, that Martin taught Physical Education both in Secondary and Further Education settings because he wanted to 'inspire and motivate others [to exercise/play sport]'.

Despite a busy lifestyle, Martin 'scheduled training and exercise into each week . . . cycling, going to the gym 3 or 4 times a week, purely just for physical activity and mental wellbeing' and described a relationship with PA that was 'very, very well formed, very well forged'.

Our approach/methods

To allow an understanding of Martin's perceptions, views, and experiences of his caring role, the constructivist paradigm was followed. It is believed that Martin's, and the other members of the research team's, reality and knowledge are socially constructed, and it was the role of the research team to understand caring from Martin's first-hand experiences.

Carer as participant, co-researcher, and author

Despite there being barriers to carers being involved in research (Malm et al., 2021), Martin, as a participant and co-researcher, was involved in the research

From physically active to physically inactive 45

process from the outset. This enabled his voice to be heard and respected (Buckner and Yeandle, 2015). It was hoped that by taking part in the research, despite the sensitivity of the topic being discussed, Martin would find it helpful to be heard (Emanuel et al., 2004) and useful to reflect on his own experiences of being his mum's carer.

Pope (2020) posited that participants as co-researchers can be an asset to a research project, particularly where there is good rapport in the team, and researchers are responsive in their research behaviours and ethical in interactions with co-researchers. Indeed, a consideration of ethics, intrinsic to constructivism due to the inclusion of the values of both the researcher(s) and the participant(s) (Guba and Lincoln, 2004), was integral to all stages of the research process. Further, reflexivity – an 'ethical notion' (Guillemin and Gillam, 2004, p. 262, emphasis in original) allowed the research team to fully embed "a disciplined practice of critically interrogating what we do, how and why we do it" (Braun and Clarke, 2022, p. 5) in all aspects of the research.

There was a consideration of boundaries in the research team (Thurairajah, 2019) and a commitment to ensuring that there were no issues around power dynamics within the research (Pettican et al., 2023). Further, Martin was provided with contact details of an external researcher should he have any concerns that he felt unable to discuss with the research team.

The methodology using triangulated data provided another safeguard against researcher bias. Further, this single case design provides a useful insight into areas where there is a lack of in-depth investigations (Horne, 2022), in this instance, a carer's relationship with PA which was both inductive and exploratory.

A qualitative multi-method approach was adopted, drawing on a combination of various qualitative methods (Mik-Meyer, 2020). Diary entry data that was longitudinal and captured prior to the planned research, with no researcher present, was analysed and used as a grounding for discussion in a first interview between Martin and the two other researchers/authors. Martin engaged in a further data task by creating an annotated timeline to mark critical moments in his carer journey. A second interview then followed to discuss this journey mapping exercise. This allowed the interview to delve into situational insights, co-constructed by Martin and the researchers. It also acted as a member checking exercise, where Martin participated in the analysis of his own experiential narrative and served as a further layer of validation and trustworthiness (as discussed by Birt et al., 2016).

Data collection

Following The Open University institutional ethical approval, Martin, as co-researcher and involved in all stages of the research, provided signed informed consent prior to the data collection phase. Martin shared extracts of his diary recorded between October 2016 and April 2018 and was involved in two interviews between March and May 2020.

The interviews involved a 'think out loud' technique where the team analysed Martin's experiences as the discussion progressed. This meant that there was no misrepresentation of Martin's experiences and Martin was able to fully contribute to the understandings and meanings he applied to his own experiences.

46 *N. Kentzer et al.*

It was decided that if, when discussing interpretations, there was a conflict of opinions, these would be reported in the findings. However, this did not occur. Both interviews were audio recorded and transcribed verbatim, and then checked by the research team.

Data analysis

Data analysis occurred concurrently with data collection, with analytical discussions conducted during the interviews, and ongoing discussions by the research team throughout the data collection period. Following transcription of the interviews and diary extracts, an inductive, iterative, and collaborative approach was taken to analyse, code and theme the data. The process outlined by Braun and Clarke (2022), described as reflexive thematic analysis, where "subjective, situated, aware and questioning" researchers are valued, was followed. The themes were discussed within the research team to enhance rigour (Silverman, 2017). Three themes were identified: lifestyle choices, loss of social and physically active self, and barriers to PA.

Analysing Martin's experience

Lifestyle choices

Following his mum suffering a severe stroke in 2016, Martin gave up his teaching role and became his mum's sole, full-time carer. This was a role he stressed was one he chose:

> because of the relationship and the love I had for my Mum, and the caring role was then my new occupation. That is how I saw it.

Making sense of an event at the very beginning of his caring role, he was asked about his own needs by a carer support agency and responded that 'I'm a physical activities person, I like to go the gym, and such and I'd like that to continue'. Even though he was keen for PA to be a part of his life in his new role, once his mum was discharged from the hospital six weeks post stroke, he 'knew it [physical activity] would be difficult, but from that moment on it began to gradually hit home'.

Martin highlighted that his 'relationship with PA changed because [his] energies were going to Mum and purely to Mum's care' and that his own health and wellbeing 'became a secondary focus'. Indeed, he reflected that:

> My own health and wellbeing wasn't my primary goal anymore and all that contradicts the fact that . . . we [carers] need to be fit and healthy. It's common sense really, it's basic logic but your basic logic and mine certainly, went out of the window because it was Mum [that was the main focus].

From physically active to physically inactive   47

Loss of social and physically active self

Isolation featured as a key barrier to Martin being physically active. Martin highlighted that his isolation went 'much deeper than' his remote location:

> Yeah the isolation was really feeling . . . that once Mum was able to come home and discharged from hospital . . . I knew it would be difficult but from that moment on it began to gradually hit home.. . . I lost all . . . all of my social network that I had from going cycling, by going to the gym . . . from being at work . . . so that was cut off.

Martin's well-developed relationship with PA prior to his mum suffering a stroke allowed him to initially find time to exercise. However, Martin noted that his motivation to engage in these activities began to diminish, despite his understanding 'that if I did exercise it may make me feel better, both physically and mentally'. He found that taking part in PA became 'increasingly difficult' and at 18 months post his mum's stroke, he noted 'having no energy to exercise' and his 'relationship with, the love and the fun I had with PA just changed and gradually depleted'.

Following a period of his own ill health, Martin described a 'feeling of guilt' when he had to move his mum into respite care when he was recovering from scarlet fever. He stated 'I should've been stronger, physically stronger and not been ill. I should've been able to look after my Mum without becoming ill and without becoming run down'. There was one positive outcome, however, to this challenging time. Martin reflected that this was a 'trigger point' where he acknowledged the importance of his own health and wellbeing, stating 'I need to go back and do something here'.

It was not until July 2019, however, two months after the respite was in place and almost three years post his mum's stroke, that he accessed his friend's garage gym once or twice a week. It took him 'a while . . . doing that . . . this [getting] over [the] feeling of guilt'.

Barriers to physical activity

In addition to the readjustment in priorities as a key factor in Martin's changing relationship with PA, there were several barriers discussed. This included guilt, a lack of energy and a feeling of being 'tired' and having 'no energy' despite knowing that he should 'make time for exercise' in his daily routine. He also lacked motivation reflecting that:

> When Mum had the stroke and particularly when Mum came home, my mindset changed, and I lacked the motivation to do exercise.

Four hours of budgeted respite support was provided from the outcome of a carer's needs assessment, with the aim 'to give me time to exercise and some time to myself'. However, 'unfortunately my time was not used for exercise; rather it was for shopping and gardening chores etc.'. More respite time, to allow for PA 'along with other domestic demands' which included cooking, housework, diabetes care and daily care (such as lifting) was 'limited by finances' and there wasn't the 'revenue to afford this option'.

There was a clear conflict evident within Martin's discourse regarding his beliefs and expectations of his caring responsibilities and his enjoyment of and need to exercise, agreeing that he did not see PA as being part of a carer's identity. This was illustrated by him highlighting the World Health Organisation's recommendations for PA and why he, despite having 'very good organisational time management skills', was unable to achieve them:

> So yes, the time practically I could have made the time available, but it was the mindset that was potentially stopping me find the time.

Discussion

Following his mum's stroke, Martin's relationships with his mum, previous colleagues, and friends changed immediately. His income and identity as a teacher were instantly lost as well as his relationship with PA. PA had previously been an integral part of who Martin was, and because of his location, his often-unconscious expectations of his caring role and his change in motivations, Martin found himself 'cut-off'. Martin was initially able to participate in PA, but this reduced quickly, and he found it increasingly difficult to engage in PA, experiencing many of the barriers reported in the literature, such as guilt, no energy, no motivation, time required for caring responsibilities and cost (Horne et al., 2021; Lindsay et al., 2023).

Like the participants in Cao et al.'s (2021) research, Martin, although having an in-depth understanding that being physically active would improve his mental and physical health, could not overcome these barriers to PA. Such was the influence of his caring role, Martin was unable to adhere to previously well-formed physical activity behaviours, despite having many of the positive correlates towards being physically active recognised by Biddle et al. (2021). These include Martin having strong social support for PA, a confidence in PA behaviours, being physically fit and having the equipment / environment to support PA.

It took Martin's own serious ill health, which required his mum to go into respite care, and the resulting guilt experienced, to make him realise that his own health was vital to him being able to care effectively for his mum. Indeed, the physical and mental health benefits gained from PA was identified as a facilitator to PA for carers by Lindsay et al. (2023). Ultimately, this increase in Martin's self-care was part of his ongoing priority to put his mum's care first. Carers prioritising others above themselves is widely reported in the literature (e.g., Carers UK, 2019; 2021; 2022).

Analysing Martin's challenging relationship with physical activity highlights the importance of understanding the complexities of the caring role when supporting carers to adopt or adhere to PA. Indeed, Michie, Atkins and West (2014) argued that a person must have capability, opportunity, and motivation to do physical activity. For a carer, therefore, this would mean knowledge and ability to be active, to be given the opportunity to be active (e.g., respite, social support) and they must want

From physically active to physically inactive 49

to be active more than they want to do any competing behaviour. Arguably Martin had the first two components, but not the third.

Drawing together theories and evidence, Mitchie and colleagues (2011; 2014) created the Behaviour Change Wheel which stressed the need for a behavioural analysis for each target population when developing a PA intervention. Given the complex findings of Martin's individual case, it is recommended that an evidence-based framework such as this, is used to develop PA interventions for carers but with consideration of the different experiences, and personal characteristics, of carers (i.e., age, gender, care recipient's condition), and not as a whole population.

Reifsteck, Gill and Brooks (2013) argue that a strong athletic identity is logically related to a strong engagement in PA, allowing Martin's experiences to be discussed within the context of existing research into athletic identity. Martin still identified with his athletic identity when he was approached by the carer support at the hospital immediately post his mum's stroke but once his mum was discharged six weeks later, he realised that this was going to change, endorsing Eifert et al.'s (2015) 'role engulfment and losing self' aspect of gaining a carer identity. Martin's expectations and practices of being his mum's carer resulted in him placing his mum's needs before his own, meaning elements of his athletic identity such as his teaching role, friendships and leisure activities immediately ceased.

Martin's experiences highlight the social context in which PA is embedded, and supports Piggin's (2020) holistic definition of PA. Further, the loss of self (both social and physically active) that Martin discusses, show how the social and physically active self are interconnected. As he lost one, he lost the other. This is reflected in research with athletes who have been forced to retire, a point at which Demetriou et al. (2020) recognised as a potential grieving period for loss of community, a loss of a sense of belonging.

Research by Yao, Laurencelle and Trudeau (2020) reported that athletic identity decreases steadily when an athlete leaves sport and becomes an ex-athlete. Carers who identify with a PA identity, therefore, need support to maintain PA in the early stages of transition to ensure that this behaviour is not lost. Lindsay et al. (2022) endorsed this claim, concluding that interventions and policies should aim to support the transition from non-carer to carer status to help establish positive PA habits. Furthermore, unlike Martin whose expectation of the caring role, often unconscious, was that PA had no place in his identity as a carer, carers could be supported to associate PA as an integral part of the caring role.

Given that Martin's physical activity was embedded with sport, it was appropriate to look at sport transition research and athletic identity. However, this will not always be the case for carers and therefore physical activity identity (Brown and Meca, 2023) could be of use for future research.

Conclusion

Examining Martin's case allowed the opportunity to explore and analyse an alternative, original perspective of the caring experience. Co-constructed research helped to develop an understanding of a carer's PA identity and is further validated by the carer, Martin, as co-researcher and author.

50 *N. Kentzer et al.*

It is recommended that further carer co-constructed research would contribute to future understandings of carer PA identities which would be valuable in supporting the implementation of future PA interventions for carers. It is important to note that in this co-constructed research, Martin is educated to Postgraduate level and so researchers must be mindful of ensuring co-researcher opportunities are accessible to all (Fraser et al., 2022).

References

Beatie, B.E. et al. (2019) 'Caregiver identity in care partners of persons living with mild cognitive impairment', *Dementia*, 20(7), pp. 2323–2339. Available at: https://doi.org/10.1177/1471301221994317.

Biddle, S. et al. (2021) *Psychology of Physical Activity: Determinants, Well-Being and Interventions*. New York: Routledge.

Birt, L. et al. (2016) 'Member checking: A tool to enhance trustworthiness or merely a nod to validation?', *Qualitative Health Research*, 26(13), pp. 1802–1811. Available at: https://doi.org/10.1177/1049732316654870.

Braun, V. and Clarke, V. (2022) *Thematic Analysis: A Practical Guide*. London: Sage Publications.

Brewer, B.W. et al. (2010) 'Self-protective changes in athletic identity following anterior cruciate ligament reconstruction', *Psychology of Sport and Exercise*, 11(1), p. 1. Available at: https://doi.org/10.1016/J.PSYCHSPORT.2009.09.005.

Brimblecombe, N. et al. (2018) 'Review of the international evidence on support for unpaid carers', *Journal of Long-Term Care*, 0(0), pp. 25–40. Available at: https://doi.org/10.31389/JLTC.3.

Brimblecombe, N. and Cartagena Farias, J. (2022) 'Inequalities in unpaid carer's health, employment status and social isolation', *Health and Social Care in the Community*, 30(6), pp. e6564–e6576. Available at: https://doi.org/10.1111/HSC.14104.

Brown, C. et al. (2018) 'Athletes' experiences of social support during their transition out of elite sport: An interpretive phenomenological analysis', *Psychology of Sport and Exercise*, 36, pp. 71–80. Available at: https://doi.org/10.1016/j.psychsport.2018.01.003.

Brown, D.M.Y. and Meca, A. (2023) 'An examination of the psychometric properties of the Exercise Identity Scale and its adaptation to physical activity', *SportRχiv*. Available at: https://doi.org/10.51224/SRXIV.172.

Buckner, L. and Yeandle, S. (2015) *Valuing Carers 2015: The Rising Value of Carers' Support*. London: Carers UK. Available at www.carersuk.org/media/5r1lcm2k/cuk-valuing-carers-2015-web.pdf (accessed 29 January 2024).

Cao, V. et al. (2010) 'Changes in activities of wives caring for their husbands following stroke', *Physiotherapy Canada*, 62(1), pp. 35–43. Available at: https://doi.org/10.3138/physio.62.1.35.

Carers UK (2019) *State of Caring: A Snapshot of Unpaid Care in the UK*. London: Carers UK. Available at: www.carersuk.org/media/khgkb3fs/state-of-caring-2019-report.pdf (accessed 29 January 2024).

Carers UK (2021) *Carers and Physical Activity: A Study of the Barriers, Motivations and Experiences of Unpaid Carers aged 55 and over in England*. London: Carers UK. Available at: www.carersuk.org/media/rr2lwmxg/carers-and-physical-activity-report.pdf (accessed 29 January 2024).

Carers UK (2022) *State of Caring 2022: A Snapshot of Unpaid Care in the UK*. London: Carers UK. Available at: www.carersuk.org/media/ew5e4swg/cuk_state_of_caring_2022_report.pdf (accessed 29 January 2024).

Carers UK (2023) *Policy Briefing: Physical Activity and Unpaid Carers in Wales*. Carers UK London. Available at: www.carersuk.org/media/ugepxids/physical-activity-policy-briefing.pdf (accessed 29 January 2024).

From physically active to physically inactive 51

Danucalov, M.A. et al. (2015) 'Yoga and compassion meditation program improve quality of life and self-compassion in family caregivers of Alzheimer's disease patients: A randomized controlled trial', *Geriatrics and Gerontology International,* 17(1), pp. 85–91. Available at: https://doi.org/10.1111/ggi.12675.

del-Pino-Casado, R. et al. (2021) 'Subjective caregiver burden and anxiety in informal caregivers: A systematic review and meta-analysis', *PLOS ONE,* 16(3), p. e0247143. Available at: https://doi.org/10.1371/JOURNAL.PONE.0247143.

Demetriou, A. et al. (2020) 'Forced retirement transition: A narrative case study of an elite Australian Rules football player', *International Journal of Sport and Exercise Psychology,* 18(3), pp. 321–335. Available at: https://doi.org/10.1080/1612197X.2018.1519839.

Eifert, E. et al. (2015) 'Family caregiver identity: A literature review', *American Journal of Health Education,* 46(6), pp. 357–367. Available at: https://doi.org/10.1080/19325037.2015.1099482.

Emanuel, E.J. et al. (2004) 'Talking with terminally ill patients and their caregivers about death, dying, and bereavement', *Archives of Internal Medicine,* 164(18), pp. 1999–2004. Available at: https://doi.org/10.1001/archinte.164.18.1999.

Fairlie, L. et al. (2019) 'Navigating the shift from netballer to former netballer: The experience of retirement from elite netball in Australia', *Sport in Society,* 23(7), pp. 1100–1118. Available at: https://doi.org/10.1080/17430437.2019.1597856.

Fraser, C. et al. (2022) 'A blueprint for involvement: Reflections of lived experience co-researchers and academic researchers on working collaboratively', *Research Involvement and Engagement,* 8(1), pp. 1–16. Available at: https://doi.org/10.1186/S40900-022-00404-3/TABLES/1.

Gibbons, S.W. et al. (2014) 'Liminality as a conceptual frame for understanding the family caregiving rite of passage: An integrative review', *Research in Nursing and Health,* 37, pp. 423–436. Available at: https://doi.org/10.1002/nur.21622.

Guba, E.G. and Lincoln, Y.S. (2004) 'Competing paradigms in qualitative research: Theories and issues', in S. Nagy Hesse-Biber and P. Levy (eds) *Approaches to Qualitative Research: A Reader on Theory and Practice.* Oxford: Oxford University Press, pp. 17–38.

Guillemin, M. and Gillam, L. (2004) 'Qualitative inquiry ethics, Reflexivity, and "ethically important moments" in research', *Qualitative Inquiry,* 10, pp. 261–280. Available at: https://doi.org/10.1177/1077800403262360.

Harris, D.L. (2020) 'Introduction', in D.L. Harris (ed.) *Non-Death Loss and Grief: Context and Clinical Implications.* London: Routledge, pp. 1–6.

Horne, J. et al. (2021) 'A systematic review on the prevalence of physical activity, and barriers and facilitators to physical activity, in informal carers in the United Kingdom', *Journal of Physical Activity and Health,* 18(2), pp. 212–218. Available at: https://doi.org/10.1123/JPAH.2020-0526.

Horne, J. (2022) 'Researching athletic development', in C. Heaney, N. Kentzer, and B. Oakley (eds) *Athletic Development: A Psychological Perspective.* London: Routledge, pp. 70–84.

Kaddour, L. and Kishita, N. (2020) 'Anxiety in informal dementia carers: A meta-analysis of prevalence', *Journal of Geriatric Psychiatry and Neurology,* 33(3), pp. 161–172. Available at: https://doi.org/10.1177/0891988719868313.

Larkin, M., Henwood, M. and Milne, A. (2019) 'Carer related research and knowledge: Findings from a scoping review', *Health and Social Care in the Community,* 27, pp. 55–67. Available at: https://doi.org/10.1111/hsc.12586.

Lindsay, R.K. et al. (2022) 'The prevalence of physical activity among informal carers: A systematic review of international literature', *Sport Sciences for Health,* 18, pp. 1071–1118. Available at: https://doi.org/10.1007/s11332-021-00893-x.

Lindsay, R.K. et al. (2023) 'Barriers and facilitators to physical activity among informal carers: A systematic review of international literature', *International Journal of Care and Caring,* 7(3), pp. 498–526. Available at: https://doi.org/10.1332/2397882 21X16746510534114.

52 N. Kentzer et al.

Lloyd, J., Patterson, T. and Muers, J. (2016) 'The positive aspects of caregiving in dementia: A critical review of the qualitative literature', *Dementia*, 15(6), pp. 1534–1561. Available at: https://doi.org/10.1177/1471301214564792/FORMAT/EPUB.

Loi, S.M. et al. (2016) 'Factors associated with depression in older carers', *International Journal of Geriatric Psychiatry*, 31(3), pp. 294–301. Available at: https://doi.org/10.1002/GPS.4323.

Lopes De Melo, A.P. et al. (2020) '"Life is taking me where I need to go": Biographical disruption and new arrangements in the lives of female family carers of children with congenital Zika syndrome in Pernambuco, Brazil', *Viruses*, 12(12), pp. 1410. Available at: https://doi.org/10.3390/v12121410.

Malewezi, E. et al. (2022) 'A different way of life: A qualitative study on the experiences of family caregivers of stroke survivors living at home', *British Journal of Community Nursing*, 27(11) pp. 558–566. Available at: https://doi.org/10.12968/bjcn.2022.27.11.558.

Malm, C. et al. (2021) 'What motivates informal carers to be actively involved in research, and what obstacles to involvement do they perceive?', *Research Involvement and Engagement*, 7(1), 80. Available at: https://doi.org/10.1186/s40900-021-00321-x.

Martis, C.S. et al. (2023) 'The effectiveness of yoga therapy on caregivers of people living with dementia: A systematic review and meta-analysis of randomized controlled trials', *Clinical Epidemiology and Global Health*, 19, 101192. Available at: https://doi.org/10.1016/J.CEGH.2022.101192.

Michie, S., Atkins, L. and West, R. (2014) *The Behaviour Change Wheel: A Guide to Designing Interventions*. Sutton: Silverback Publishing.

Michie, S., van Stralen, M.M. and West, R. (2011) 'The behaviour change wheel: A new method for characterising and designing behaviour change interventions', *Implementation Science*, 6(1), 42. Available at: https://doi.org/10.1186/1748-5908-6-42.

Mik-Meyer, N. (2020) 'Multimethod qualitative research', in D. Silverman (ed.) *Qualitative Research*. London: Sage, pp. 357–374.

Montgomery, R. and Kosloski, K. (2009) 'Caregiving as a process of changing identity: Implications for caregiver support', *Generations*, 33(1), pp. 47–52.

OECD (2019) *Health at a Glance 2019: OECD Indicators*. Paris: Organisation for Economic Co-operation and Development Publishing. Available at: https://doi.org/10.1787/4DD50C09-EN.

Petrillo, M. and Bennett, M. (2022) *Valuing Carers 2021: England and Wales*. London: Carers UK/Centre for Care. Available at: https://centreforcare.ac.uk/wp-content/uploads/2023/05/Valuing_Carers_WEB2.pdf (accessed 29 January 2024).

Pettican, A. et al. (2023) 'Doing together: Reflections on facilitating the co-production of participatory action research with marginalised populations', *Qualitative Research in Sport, Exercise and Health*, 15(2), pp. 202–219. Available at: https://doi.org/10.1080/2159676X.2022.2146164.

Piggin, J. (2020) 'What is physical activity? A holistic definition for teachers, researchers and policy makers', *Frontiers in Sports and Active Living*, 2, 532524. Available at: https://doi.org/10.3389/FSPOR.2020.00072.

Pope, E.M. (2020) 'From participants to co-researchers: Methodological alterations to a qualitative case study', *The Qualitative Report*, 25(10), pp. 3749–3761. Available at: https://doi.org/10.46743/2160-3715/2020.4394.

Reifsteck, E.J., Gill, D.L. and Brooks, D.L. (2013) 'The relationship between athletic identity and physical activity among former college athletes', *Athletic Insight*, 5(3), pp. 271–284.

Ross, A. et al. (2020) 'Factors that influence health-promoting behaviors in cancer caregivers', *Oncology Nursing Forum*, 47(6), pp. 692–702. Available at: https://doi.org/10.1188/20.ONF.692-702.

Saban, K.L. and Hogan, N.S. (2012) 'Female caregivers of stroke survivors: Coping and adapting to a life that once was', *Journal of Neuroscience Nursing*, 44(1), pp. 2–14. Available at: https://doi.org/10.1097/JNN.0b013e31823ae4f9.

From physically active to physically inactive 53

Sanders, G. and Stevinson, C. (2017) 'Associations between retirement reasons, chronic pain, athletic identity, and depressive symptoms among former professional footballers', *European Journal of Sport Science*, 17(10), pp. 1311–1318. Available at: https://doi.org/ 10.1080/17461391.2017.1371795.

Silverman, D. (2017) 'How was it for you? The Interview Society and the irresistible rise of the (poorly analyzed) interview', *Qualitative Research*, 17(2), pp. 144–158. Available at: https://doi.org/10.1177/1468794116668231.

Stambulova, N.B., Ryba, T.V. and Henriksen, K. (2021) 'Career development and transitions of athletes: The International Society of Sport Psychology Position Stand Revisited', *International Journal of Sport and Exercise Psychology*, 19(4) pp. 524–550. Available at: https://doi.org/10.1080/1612197X.2020.1737836.

Thurairajah, K. (2019) 'Uncloaking the researcher: Boundaries in qualitative research', *Qualitative Sociology Review*, 15(1), pp. 132–147. Available at: https://doi.org/10.18778/1733-8077.15.1.06.

WHO (2010) *Global Recommendations on Physical Activity for Health*. Geneva: World Health Organisation.

WHO (2020) *WHO Guidelines on Physical Activity and Sedentary Behaviour*. Geneva: World Health Organisation.

WHO (2022) *Global Status Report on Physical Activity 2022*. Geneva: World Health Organisation.

Willis, P., Vickery, A. and Symonds, J. (2020) '"You have got to get off your backside; otherwise, you'll never get out": Older male carers' experiences of loneliness and social isolation', *International Journal of Care and Caring*, 4(3), pp. 311–330. Available at: https://doi.org/10.1332/239788220X15912928956778.

Yao, P.L., Laurencelle, L. and Trudeau, F. (2020) 'Former athletes' lifestyle and self-definition changes after retirement from sports', *Journal of Sport and Health Science*, 9(4), pp. 376–383. Available at: https://doi.org/10.1016/J.JSHS.2018.08.006.

5 Both sides of the coin

A mother's experience of caring for an adult daughter living with serious life-limiting illness

Susan Walker

Introduction

This chapter offers reflections from the lived experience of a mother who has recently transitioned into the role of live-in carer for her adult daughter who is coping with life after leukaemia, together with a separate ongoing life-limiting medical condition. The daughter's life expectancy is not overly long. The disruption of the mother's biographical trajectory has entailed a number of losses including that of an expected future in paid employment, independent housing in a familiar location and the ability to make long term plans for most aspects of life. This is described as a form of disenfranchised grief which is not readily acknowledged by society at large.

However, the mother attests to many positive aspects of caregiving that she has experienced including the life-affirming relational dynamic of two adults sharing life together, an emerging sense of new meaning and purpose, and the feeling that this experience is both a natural rite of passage and a privilege. In addition to documenting a carer's experience of revising taken-for-granted meanings in the light of their changed social world, the mother's narrative resonates with Meaning Reconstruction Theory and the Dual Process Model of Grief. A holistic picture of caregiving is offered.

Biographical expectations

It's often said that life is a journey: we set off, we travel in a certain direction and eventually we get somewhere. For most people, at least in the UK, the expected trajectory is something like this: we're born, we go to school, perhaps university, we get a job, a house, a social life, we pursue our career, we save for our pension with the hope of a secure and interesting retirement. Along the way, some of us fall in love, settle down and have children. We anticipate that our children will grow up and go their merry way into adult lives of their own whilst our role as parent will fade somewhat into the background. We foresee our former parental duty of hands-on care morphing into something less active, though still supportive. From here on in we will be much more in the background of our children's lives, as they will be busy pursuing their own career, social life and, possibly, family life. Now

DOI: 10.4324/9781003435365-5

Both sides of the coin 55

our contribution will consist of making occasional, pleasurable visits to their home, being invited to share in celebrations and perhaps holidays and enjoying a pleasant correspondence via phone, email, Facetime and so on. Recent research from the Office for National Statistics supports the argument that something similar to the route outlined above is normative (ONS, 2019a; ONS, 2019b).

Obviously, there will be deviations from the norm, but for many people, including myself, later life will be perceived as the point at which there is time to enjoy that retirement we saved for. Maybe we'll book a cruise, take a geriatric gap year and visit gorillas in Uganda, seriously update our salsa dancing skills or build a house by the sea. Finally, we have time on our hands and the means to indulge some pleasant extravagances or to happily do nothing very much. Laslett (1996) purports that being free from the constraints of work and family, at this stage, people can pursue whatever constitutes for them a good quality of life. Similarly, Higgs et al. (2009) note that many now conceptualise later life as a time of adventure, personal growth and fulfilment after a lifetime of work.

Becoming a carer

As I reflect on my own life journey, I note that it has recently deviated somewhat from the norm described and has taken a rather unexpected diversion. Now in my early 60s, instead of existing in the background of my 32-year-old daughter's world, as I happily wind down towards retirement, I find that I have relocated my entire life to become her live-in carer, as she negotiates life after leukaemia on the background of a separate ongoing life-limiting medical condition. I made these radical changes to my life in rather dramatic circumstances. Within hours of being diagnosed with leukaemia, my daughter was admitted to hospital to begin intensive treatment which would entail a lengthy in-patient hospital stay, emergency surgery and a spell on the intensive care unit, followed by months of further demanding treatment as an out-patient. She faced all this as a single woman, living 200 miles away from family and at the height of the Covid-19 pandemic. Without hesitation, I travelled to the hospital and arranged temporary accommodation for myself nearby in order to support her through her illness.

Then, as it became clear that, from this point forward, my daughter would need ongoing support with her life, and that her life expectancy may not be overly long, I decided to relocate permanently to the place where she had established her adult life and work. This move involved selling my house, leaving my job and the location I had called home for many years, which was replete with friends and family. My daughter and I bought a house together and I found part-time work which fitted in around her support needs. I now spend much of my day engaged in helping her with personal care; with domestic duties such as cooking, cleaning, laundry and shopping; managing household finances and driving my daughter to her work, various medical appointments and social engagements. In short, I had become one of the reportedly 6.5 million unpaid informal carers in the UK (Eurofound, 2022). An informal carer may be defined as anyone who cares, unpaid, for a friend or family

56   S. Walker

member who due to illness, disability, a mental health problem or an addiction, cannot cope without their support (Carers Trust, 2022).

Though at times challenging and certainly different from how I have lived in recent times, in many ways, life is good. It is both a pleasure and a privilege to share in my daughter's life in such intimate ways and to connect with her at such a deep level. However, the dissimilarities between expectations I had for life in my early 60s and how things have turned out should not be underplayed. Whilst I relished the years spent at home with my children when they were pre-schoolers, I never imagined that I would spend these years in such close quarters with one of them and in such a caring role. The predicted arc of my life has been significantly disrupted.

Loss and grief encountered as a carer

There is no doubt that the disruption of my expected biographical trajectory entailed a number of losses including that of an expected future in paid employment, the loss of independent housing in a familiar location and the ability to make long-term plans for most aspects of life including social life, companionship and holidays. Losses of this kind clearly entailed considerable changes in my life and, at first, I was puzzled as to how to respond to the enormity of my situation and the suddenness by which it had come upon me. Others around me, including my employer and some family members and friends also seemed to falter in knowing what to say to me. I wondered whether people failed to perceive that I was encountering loss; after all, there had not been a death. Thankfully, my daughter had not died and yet her life had changed irrevocably, and major adjustments would now have to be made in both our lives. Moreover, such adjustments were suffused with poignancy. As I look back and reflect on this, I have come to regard this period as a form of disenfranchised grief, that is grief which is not really acknowledged or recognised by society at large (Doka, 1989).

It could seem strange, exaggerated or even disrespectful to talk of changes in my life circumstances as being co-terminus with grief. It could be asserted that the concept of grief in relation to death is so well-founded that the term 'grief' should be reserved for the period of bereavement and mourning which normally follows the profound and very real separation that death brings. Indeed, many would agree with Bowlby and others that grief is the appropriate response to the breaking of significant attachment bonds (Bowlby, 1980; Jordan, 2020).

However, recent years have seen a growing recognition that there are many non-death losses experienced in life which provoke a process akin to grieving with its attendant psychological shock, emotional pain and the unwelcome necessity of making major adjustments in how life is now to be lived in response to the new status quo. Examples of such losses include the loss of employment, the loss of a partner through relationship break up, the loss of housing, and the loss of physical or mental capacity due to illness or accident. These kinds of losses are neither trivial nor transient but represent times of considerable emotional and psychological pain and social dislocation and have the potential to evoke a type of grief reaction. Harris (2019) purports that grieving is a basic human instinctual response to all types of losses, not just to death. This is partly because the losses, such as the ones I have described, concern core aspects of a person's assumptive world and changes at this level touch on issues around meaning and purpose.

On the other hand, it is questionable whether every loss experienced in life can be described as grief-triggering. Some losses, though evoking intense emotions at the time, are transitory and do not touch on existential matters. For example, some media accounts of the public's responses to the various lockdowns caused by the Covid-19 pandemic, though redolent with the rhetoric of grief, were not of lasting import. For example, Gottlieb commented that people were grieving cancelled celebrations and sporting events (Gottlieb, 2020) and Kessler, whose seminal work with Kubler-Ross gave the world the five stages of grief model, argued that the pandemic was forcing people to experience a number of different griefs (Berinato, 2020). Often the losses cited were temporary, such as being prevented from attending family gatherings, taking part in pleasurable pastimes such as team sports or making visits to favourite places. These losses were not related to core aspects of people's worlds and the activities allegedly lost would be resumed at some future time.

My situation was altogether different in type, characterised by permanence and existential matters. Firstly, it concerned key aspects of my life: where I would live, what job I could now logistically take on in order to earn my living and what primary role would my life now entail. Former patterns of life could not, and would not, be returned to. Inevitably, new patterns would have to be established and as new roles for my life emerged, new meanings would have to be grappled with and understood by myself and others. I was in the process of transitioning from being known as an independent leader of a faith community to becoming a live-in carer. Within this scenario, the object of my grief was not a person, but my former life. I was grieving the loss of various possibilities for my life (Ratcliffe, 2022) and, moreover, possibilities which were indicative of the basic structure of a certain kind of life, which would now be impossible to pursue.

All of this became crystallised for me during a seemingly mundane occurrence at my new house. Having sold my former home, my daughter and I bought a house together and the day came for my furniture to arrive. As my daughter's leukaemia treatment had taken place during the Covid-19 pandemic, with its attendant restrictions on movement around the country, all my furniture and possessions had to be packed up by others and sent north to my new home via a removal company. I had not physically seen these items for over a year. As I sat amongst the packing boxes and scattered pieces of well-loved furniture, I was suddenly overcome by a wave of emotion which swept over me with surprising power. I felt my heart-rate increase, my breathing quicken and I had to sit down. I could utter no words, but to my chagrin, tears came into my eyes and I felt quite overwhelmed. For a good while, all I could do was to sit still and stare. Later that night I wrote about this episode in my journal, and I noted that I felt a little ashamed to be crying over mere material possessions:

> What are things compared to everything that J's been through and what are they to cry about when you have this chance to be such an important part of the next stage of her life? Get a grip woman! This is a good day not a sad one. Then why was I so knocked for six? The only thing I can compare this

58 *S. Walker*

to is the once or twice after my mother died when I was caught unawares by a sudden surge of . . . something . . . so much so that I was stopped in my tracks. The time when I saw someone wearing one of her M&S skirts and my heart skipped a beat (and not in a good way) and the time I was powerless to move away from her favourite cake on the supermarket shelf. Rationally, those incidents didn't make a lot of sense either, but I knew they were part of my grieving. I knew it was to do with having to accept that my mother was gone and that, for me, life would never be the same again. Is that it? Is this just me acknowledging that there's no turning back now: I've really sold the house in the midlands and made this permanent move to the north east to be with J; I've really left my job to commit to this life here? Maybe I'm still in the process of letting go of some of this stuff. These are massive life changes: no wonder it felt like a sort of shockwave. Maybe that's normal?

And so, this seemingly unconnected incident served to communicate to me that I could be undergoing a grief-type reaction to the enormity of everything that had taken place during the past year or so and to the changes yet to come. Perhaps bizarrely, my furniture served as a symbol of my grief.

Interestingly, once I had started to accept that I might be in the midst of the chaos of grieving for my former life, I was able to think about finding a way to navigate through the disarray. I wondered whether my sort of experience was a common one amongst those who were plunged unexpectedly into the caring role and whether I would benefit from connecting with such people. I hoped to access some communal wisdom that would at least affirm my grieving and perhaps suggest possible ways forward.

I applied to join a Carer Support Group at the local cancer support centre. I thought this would be a good choice as my daughter was attending this centre's Young Women with Cancer Support Group and she was finding the experience extremely helpful. However, I was turned down by the Carer Group organiser because my daughter was apparently 'not sick enough yet'. The problem was that all the other carers in the group had associated care recipients who were now terminally ill, and it was deemed that my presence within the group would not be welcome because my daughter was in remission. The centre could not offer me a more appropriate group at that time. It is possible that a set of carers who were in a similar position to myself would have welcomed my engagement with their group. As things stood, I was left feeling somewhat abandoned. Whilst I had no desire to add to others' difficulties, I needed support NOW to make necessary psychological and social adjustments, but instead I began to wonder whether what I had identified as grief was even worthy of professional and societal attention.

Attig (2004) pointed out that the way in which one's grief is treated can be shaped according to another's assumptions of what this should consist of and how it should look. According to Doka (1989), social support and validation is withheld from the grieving individual because their loss is not viewed as warranting grief. At this point, it certainly felt like the grief-like feelings I was attempting to negotiate were not sanctioned, at least not by the cancer support centre. Gitterman and

Knight (2019) noted that grieving for the non-death losses of one's place and all that is familiar, together with associated opportunities, can go largely unnoticed in society. Consequently, there are often limited outlets for such grieving (Packman et al., 2014), which results in people being left on their own to grieve and suffer from these types of non-death losses. Dominguez (2018) also noted that disenfranchised grief can be a lonely experience, as disconnecting is an overarching characteristic of this phenomenon.

Without doubt, my confidence to reach out for help from external agencies had been undermined and there was a real risk that I would withdraw into myself with my muddled feelings. However, rather than withdrawing into isolation, I decided to view this incident as merely my first attempt at accessing support and I persisted in exploring other avenues of help which would afford connection and community. This led to the development of a more positive outlook on my situation.

Dealing with loss in the caring role: Finding the positives

One of the first helpful things I did to ensure I was connected into a helpful network was to join a fellowship group at my new church. This meant that I went to someone's home once a week to meet up with around ten people for prayer, bible study and general socialising. Additionally, I made a point of having regular supportive phone and video calls with friends and family where I could offload and reflect with others on all that was happening in my life or where I could simply enjoy the company of other people.

My church fellowship group not only provided sympathetic and spiritual support but also turned out to be a very sociable space; they often had gatherings with food, drink and fun and I found that being able to participate in such events felt like taking a breath of fresh air. Similarly, listening to the ups and downs of the everyday lives of friends and family had the power to transport me away from my own worries and propel me into the larger space of social normality where my life related to and intertwined with others and did not exclusively revolve around my caring duties. Undoubtedly, my life was not what it had once been, but it seemed as if I was starting to see the next portion of it as imbued with all kinds of positive possibilities. Harris (2019) has described this kind of thinking as a reweaving process which incorporates the new experiences into the overarching narrative of one's life, the purpose of which is to make one's world coherent once more. I would add to this that such a reweaving process has the potential to cast a constructive light on the new experiences encountered and those which lie ahead.

One of the most positive aspects of my new situation was being able to spend time with my daughter every day by virtue of sharing accommodation with her. This meant our relationship could grow in new and deep ways hitherto unforeseen. The fact that we had set up home together, as opposed to her 'coming home to mum's house to be looked after', was significant. If she had 'come home' there could have been a sense of dependency, but two adults choosing to live together presupposes a different kind of relational dynamic, which is more about co-dependency and mutuality, with no dominant power differential. This is perhaps well-illustrated in what may seem like a trivial matter, that is the process of choosing fittings and furnishings for our new home. Many robust discussions were had regarding which pieces of furniture from our respective homes were going to make it into the new house and which were not. We agreed that the guiding principle should be an assessment of what would meet our *joint* current and future needs. We deliberately tried to look forward and not back as we built a new home which would reflect our new mode of living. It soon became very clear that in her young adulthood my daughter had developed her own aesthetic sensibilities which were sometimes at odds with mine. Nevertheless, I rejoiced in this new insight into her life and we both enjoyed the vigorous process of two equals stating their personal views.

In these and many other ways we were getting to know each other as two adults, not as parent and child. Whilst we each had our own circle of friends and were careful to give each other space, we socialised together a lot, attended the same church and made joint decisions on many day-to-day household matters such as setting the budget and deciding what to eat. Living in the same house day by day also afforded many opportunities for a deep sharing of our hopes and dreams, which would not have happened in the same way had we been living separately. To put it succinctly, we grew closer. To my everlasting joy, I found that I very much enjoyed living with the younger generation; I found my daughter's different outlook on life refreshing and infinitely interesting. I rejoiced in being, at times, the wise old woman and at others a source of amusement with my apparently archaic attitudes and language.

As time went by, I noticed a growing sense of satisfaction deep within me. I would argue that this was not just because I was able to meet my daughter's support needs. In addition to that, I sensed that the close relationship we were building with each other was beneficial to both of us. My experience is in keeping with other carers who have noted that mutuality within a caregiving dyadic relationship can generate a sense of personal accomplishment and gratification (Wang et al., 2022). Furthermore, some studies have reported that conceptualising caregiving as something constructive can have a helpful impact on the caregivers' quality of life and wellbeing (Johansson et al., 2022; Morimoto and Takebayashi, 2021). That is not to say that I had cast aside the unfortunate reason that had thrown us together, but the fact that I thoroughly enjoyed relating to my daughter as an adult and found her insights and outlook on life endlessly fascinating, seemed to carry me through the sad times.

Conceptualising myself as a carer was a significant step in this new chapter of my life. As I began to meet people in my new neighbourhood, it was necessary to find an answer to such questions as 'What do you do?' 'Are you retired?'. Without hesitation, I was happy to explain that I was my daughter's live-in carer because it seemed very clear to me that this was my new purpose in life. However, it would be disingenuous not to note that I also found a way to keep working for one flexible day a week, which allowed me to continue to use my professional skills as a Christian minister.

Notwithstanding that, the sense of purpose engendered in becoming J's carer meant that my life, as it was now, had direction and meaning. There was a job to be done and I was doing it. I have always found this notion in and of itself quite satisfying. I suspect I am what some organisational psychologists would call a

Both sides of the coin 61

'completer-finisher' (Jeanes, 2019), in that if there is a task to be done, I rejoice in the sense of having completed it to the required standard. Similarly, in becoming a carer I was required to master new skills and to overcome daily challenges which could range from working out how to get my daughter in and out of the shower safely, how to negotiate the online disability benefits system (so labyrinthine as to baffle even the most astute minotaur), to what to do on days when I was unwell.

This sense of purpose was highly motivating and helped me to persevere on difficult days and, in general, this encouraged me to actively manage my situation in terms of setting achievable goals. Furthermore, I believe it helped foster a sense of perspective; that is to not become overly stressed about every small hurdle but to aim for a more balanced approach to the role. For example, if there was a difference of opinion between my daughter and myself regarding care objectives for the day, I learned that it was important to occasionally agree to let some care tasks slide in order to allow my daughter some freedom to engage in social activity. Likewise, I schooled myself to be as patient as humanly possible with the GP receptionists who seemed to never understand the urgency of my requests. Such self-conscious coping strategies helped me to feel positive about how well I was doing as a carer, which in turn fuelled my optimism about the road ahead. Similar observations have been noted amongst those caring for people with dementia and stroke (Polenick et al., 2019; Mackenzie and Greenwood, 2012).

Another positive aspect of this experience of caring for my daughter at this time in her life is the sense that this is a kind of natural rite of passage. This was so clear to me as I talked with friends and wrote about it in my journal:

In some ways caring for J is an easy role to fulfil . . . no, not easy but natural: I'm her mother – I oversaw her coming into the world, her childhood, her growing up and leaving home and now I will oversee the final period of her life. What a privilege! I've noticed that many other mums 'get this' instantly and that's gratifying. Plus, lots of my contemporaries are busy with grandchildren – doing the physical caring, feeding, taxi-ing etc. This is my grandmother time – after all it's a bit like having J all over again and in a way that's true for both of us. Good job we were always good pals.

Some studies have noted a similar notion amongst adult children caring for aging relatives. It has been argued that, in the Asian-context, informal caregiving is often viewed as an opportunity to demonstrate what is termed 'filial piety'. This term derives from the Confucian belief that it is one's responsibility to take care of family members, and this view is purportedly fairly prevalent among Asian caregivers, particularly those with Chinese heritage (Hashimoto and Ikels, 2005; Yuan et al., 2023). However, this may not be so culturally specific; I would argue that my motivation to care for my daughter comes from comparable values. My own Christian faith enjoins believers to demonstrate the unconditional love of God in every sphere of life, including that of caring for family members. Certainly, my faith sustains me in my caregiving role and refreshes my innermost being, providing strength to continue and hope for the ultimate future for both my daughter and myself.

62   *S. Walker*

This aligns with the well-established psychological idea that having some sort of higher purpose can keep a person focused on attaining their valued goals (McKnight and Kashdan, 2009). This was classically and eloquently discussed by Frankl who, reflecting on his terrible experience in Nazi concentration camps, noticed that prisoners who could discern a sense of purpose in life were able to survive longer than those who could not (Frankl, 1959). Polenick et al. (2019) assert that having a sense of a higher purpose positively motivates informal carers to provide care and to persevere despite obstacles and difficulties. Of course, having a sense of higher purpose may affect how caregivers, such as myself, appraise our caregiving experiences; we may be more likely to view our situations in a more positive light than others (Yu et al., 2016). Nevertheless, I do not believe this negates the accuracy of my perception that there are constructive encounters to be had as a carer.

Both sides of the coin

The reflections offered in this chapter, on my unanticipated and rapid transition into the carer role, have exhibited a definite narrative quality. It is only as I look back that I find I largely achieved this through making good use of my existing personal journal; I spontaneously and naturally wrote about my situation as it unfolded. As a social scientist who has previously written about loss and grief it was then but a small step to think about these personal reflections with a more professional eye in the hope that this writing might inform the work of practitioners engaged in supporting people who are going through similar experiences.

Accordingly, I have told my tale and, in so doing, have constructed a life story that I can understand and one which I believe captures something of the person I now am. Such an approach has much in common with a Meaning Reconstruction Theory approach whereby a self-narrative is seen as an aid to making sense of a post-loss life (Neimeyer, 2016). I would not go so far as to say that I had made some sort of effortful attempt to reconfigure a viable concept of who I am and what the social world now represents for me (Neimeyer, 2001). I did not set out to reconstruct my life story but, finding myself assailed by an unexpected turn of events, I was certainly faced with the task of revising taken-for-granted meanings in order to respond realistically to my now significantly changed world (Neimeyer and Anderson, 2002).

At the beginning of this chapter, I described my life as a journey which has taken an unexpected diversion; these reflections represent the process of finding a new orientation which will help me find my way from this point forward. I have deliberately highlighted both the negative and positive ways that my life trajectory has been impacted. I have acknowledged a certain sense of loss as there have been substantial changes in my life and personal circumstances and at the same time have described how I have come to appreciate new meanings and a new sense of purpose.

In some ways this resonates with Stroebe and Shut's (1999) Dual Process of Grief Model whereby at times the bereaved person is largely loss-orientated and at others restoration-orientated, with the journey through grief being not necessarily linear. At times I still think about aspects of my life which are now lost to me but, on the whole, I choose to frame the narrative in an optimistic light. Day by day my life is being enriched far more than diminished and what I gain far outweighs anything I may have lost. Largely, I view this as merely the next chapter of my life unfolding in the myriad and mysterious ways that life always does.

I believe I have offered a holistic picture of this mother's experience of caring for my adult daughter who lives with serious life-limiting illness. I acknowledge a number of negative aspects associated with loss whilst also presenting the many positive aspects of my life as a carer. There are always two sides to the coin.

References

Attig, T. (2004) 'Disenfranchised grief revisited: Discounting hope and love', *OMEGA–Journal of Death and Dying*, 49(3), pp. 197–215. Available at: https://doi.org/10.2190/P4TT-J3BF-KFDR-5JB1.

Berinato, S. (2020) 'That discomfort you're feeling is grief', *Harvard Business Review*. Available at: https://hbr.org/2020/03/that-discomfort-youre-feeling-is-grief (accessed 14 May 2023).

Bowlby, J. (1980) *Attachment and Loss* – Volume 3: *Loss, Sadness and Depression*. New York: Basic Books.

Carers Trust (2022) *About Caring*. Available at: https://carers.org/about-caring/about-caring (accessed 14 May 2023).

Doka, K.J. (1989) 'Disenfranchised grief' in K.J. Doka (ed.) *Disenfranchised Grief: Recognizing Hidden Sorrow*. Lexington, MA: Lexington Books, pp. 3–11.

Dominguez, K.M. (2018) 'Encountering disenfranchised grief: An Investigation of the clinical lived experiences in dance/movement therapy' *American Journal of Dance Therapy*, 40, pp. 254–276. Available at: https://doi.org/10.1007/s10465-018-9281-9.

Eurofound (2022) *European Quality of Life Survey*. Dublin, Ireland: European Foundation for the Improvement of Living and Working Conditions. Available at: www.eurofound.europa.eu/data/european-quality-of-life-survey (accessed 14 May 2023).

Frankl, V. (1959) *Man's Search for Meaning*. London: Hodder and Stoughton.

Gitterman, A. and Knight, C. (2019) 'Non-death loss: Grieving for the loss of familiar place and for precious time and associated opportunities', *Clinical Social Work Journal*, 47, pp. 147–155. Available at: https://doi.org/10.1007/s10615-018-0682-5.

Gottlieb, L. (2020) 'Grieving the losses of coronavirus', *New York Times*, March 23. Available at: www.nytimes.com/2020/03/23/well/family/coronavirus-grief-loss.html (accessed 14 May 2023).

Harris, D.L. (2019) *Non-death Loss and Grief: Context and Clinical Implications*. London: Routledge.

Hashimoto, A. and Ikels, C. (2005) 'Filial piety in changing Asian societies', in M.L. Johnson (ed.) *The Cambridge Handbook of Age and Ageing*. Cambridge, UK: Cambridge University Press.

Higgs, P.F. et al. (2009) 'From passive to active consumers? Later life consumption in the UK from 1968–2005', *The Sociological Review*, 57(1), pp. 102–124. Available at: https://doi.org/10.1111/j.1467-954X.2008.01806.x.

Jeanes, E. (2019) *A Dictionary of Organizational Behaviour*. Oxford, UK: Oxford University Press. Available at: www.oxfordreference.com/display/10.1093/acref/9780191843273.001.0001/acref-9780191843273-e-35;jsessionid=1ED349611CF5253EF84F97AFBED9BA64 (accessed 2 May 2023).

Johansson, M.F. et al. (2022) 'Negative impact and positive value of caregiving in spouse carers of persons with dementia in Sweden', *International Journal of Environmental Research and Public Health*, 19(3), p. 1788. Available at: https://doi:10.3390/ijerph19031788.

64   S. Walker

Jordan, J.R. (2020) 'Lessons learned: Forty years of clinical work with suicide loss Survivors', *Frontiers in Psychology*, 11, p. 766. Available at: https://doi.org/10.3389/fpsyg.2020.00766.

Laslett, P. (1996) *A Fresh Map of Life: The Emergence of the Third Age*, 2nd edition. London: Macmillan.

Mackenzie, A. and Greenwood, N. (2012) 'Positive experiences of caregiving in stroke: A systematic review', *Disability and Rehabilitation*, 34, pp. 1413–1422. Available at: httpp://doi:10.3109/09638288.2011.650307.

McKnight, P.E. and Kashdan, T.B. (2009) 'Purpose in life as a system that creates and sustains health and well-being: An integrative, testable theory', *Review of General Psychology*, 13(3), pp. 242–251. Available at: https://doi.org/10.1037/a0017152.

Morimoto, H. and Takebayashi, Y. (2021) 'Antecedents and outcomes of enrichment among working family caregivers of people with dementia: A longitudinal analysis', *The Journals of Gerontology Series B: Psychological Sciences and Social Sciences*, 76, pp. 1060–1070. Available at: https://doi:10.1093/geronb/gbaa183.

Neimeyer, R.A. (2001) 'The language of loss: Grief therapy as a process of meaning reconstruction' in R.A. Neimeyer (ed.) *Meaning Reconstruction and the Experience of Loss*. Washington, DC: American Psychological Association, pp. 261–292.

Neimeyer, R.A. (2016) 'Meaning reconstruction in the wake of loss: Evolution of a research program', *Behaviour Change*, 33(2), pp. 65–79. Available at: https://doi.org/10.1017/bec.2016.4

Neimeyer, R.A. and Anderson, A. (2002) 'Meaning reconstruction theory', in N. Thompson, (ed.) *Loss and Grief*. Basingstoke: Palgrave, pp. 44–64.

ONS (2019a) *Milestones: Journeying into Adulthood*. London: Office for National Statistics. Available at: www.ons.gov.uk/peoplepopulationandcommunity/populationandmigration/populationestimates/articles/milestonesjourneyingintoadulthood/2019-02-18   (accessed 24 July 2023).

ONS (2019b) *Milestones: Journeying through Adulthood*. London: Office for National Statistics. Available at: www.ons.gov.uk/peoplepopulationandcommunity/populationandmigration/populationestimates/articles/milestonesjourneyingthroughadulthood/2019-12-17 (accessed 24 July 2023).

Packman, W. et al. (2014) 'Online survey as empathic bridging for the disenfranchised grief of pet loss', *OMEGA – Journal of Death and Dying*, 69(4), pp. 333–356. Available at: https://doi.org/10.2190/OM.69.4.a.

Polenick, C.A. et al. (2019) 'Purpose in life among family care partners managing dementia: Links to caregiving gains', *Gerontologist*, 59(5), pp. 424–432. Available at: https://doi:10.1093/geront/gny063.

Ratcliffe, M. (2022) *Grief Worlds*. Cambridge, MA: MIT Press.

Stroebe, M. and Shut, H. (1999) 'The dual process model of coping with bereavement: Rationale and description', *Death Studies* 23(3), pp. 197–204.

Wang, J. et al. (2022) 'The positive aspects of caregiving in dementia: A scoping review and bibliometric analysis', *Frontiers in Public Health*, 10, 985391. Available at: https://doi:10.3389/fpubh.2022.985391.

Yu, H. et al. (2016) 'Caregiving burden and gain among adult-child caregivers caring for parents with dementia in China: The partial mediating role of reciprocal filial piety' *International Psychogeriatrics*, 28(11), pp. 1845–1855. Available at: https://doi.org/10.1017/S1041610216000685.

Yuan, Q. et al. (2023). 'Positive aspects of caregiving among informal caregivers of persons with dementia in the Asian context: A qualitative study', *BMC Geriatrics,* 23(51), pp. 1–11. Available at: https://doi.org/10.1186/s12877-023-03767-8.

6 'God hasn't given up on them'

Christian dementia carers' narratives of experiencing and challenging 'anticipatory grief' and 'social death'

Jennifer Riley and John Swinton

Introduction

Dementia is 'an umbrella term for several diseases affecting memory, other cognitive abilities and behaviour that interfere significantly with a person's ability to maintain their activities of daily living' (World Health Organisation; WHO, 2024) including Alzheimer's Disease. Incidences are increasing rapidly in the UK and globally (WHO, 2024; Alzheimer's Society, 2014). Caring for people living with dementia and their carers is therefore a significant current social concern (Farrow et al., 2018) spanning multiple social domains, including: home, residential and hospice care (Fahey-McCarthy et al., 2009; Goh et al., 2022); healthcare (Cashin et al., 2019); law enforcement (Powers et al., 2020); and social work (Collins et al., 2007). Such care has many forms and sources, including organisations – not least religious communities such as Christian churches (Kevern and Walker, 2013; Friedrich, Woods and Williams, 2021; Gore et al., 2022).

Twinning practical theology and death studies scholarship and approaches, this chapter draws upon interviews with people living with dementia, their carers, and Christian theological educators. Following a theoretical background and brief methodology, it highlights both the grief, social change and challenges interviewees associated with dementia, and their desire – not least on account of their faith – to resist suggestions that those living with dementia are lost, insignificant or spiritually or socially 'dead' or 'dying'. This suggests that supporting dementia carers requires willingness to dwell simultaneously in two seemingly incompatible spaces: while responding caringly to 'anticipatory grief' and 'social death' which do – often painfully – take place, churches should also affirm the value, agency and social significance of people living with dementia.

Background

Death studies scholarship differentiates between physical death and social death, which do not occur simultaneously. As Davies (2015; 2017) highlights, where people are 'kept alive' and maintained in social networks through memories, objects or their online presence, social death may occur long after physical death. The converse also occurs; as Brannelly (2011) explains, individuals may socially die, or be

DOI: 10.4324/9781003435365-6

66   J. Riley and J. Swinton

treated as though socially dead, or 'unworthy of social participation', before their physical death. She notes that '[s]ome marginalized groups are more susceptible to this treatment than others, and one such group is people with dementia' (p. 662).

Correspondingly, dementia carers' experiences are commonly allied to 'anticipatory grief'. Lindemann (1963 [1944], p.18), a psychiatrist, coined this now widely cited term to describe military wives who, anticipating that their husbands would not return, did their 'grief work . . . so effectively' that their relationship could not be rekindled. As Moon (2016, p. 417) summarises, the women had 'psychoemotionally relinquish[ed] [their] marital relationship'. While some argue that anticipatory grief lacks conceptual clarity, and thus practical utility (Moon, 2016), others consider it a versatile tool and idiom. For example, Garand et al. (2012, p. 2) use it to explore people's experiences of what they consider 'normal bereavement in advance of the loss of a significant person', observing that that carers of people with Alzheimer's Disease experienced 'difficulty functioning' and 'missing the person they once knew' (p. 2). This highlights that anticipatory grief both anticipates future loss (physical death) and acknowledges loss(es) already in progress (changes in personality, activity and embodiment of the person as they were before developing dementia). Relatedly, Pérez-González, Vilajoana-Celaya and Guàrdia-Olmos (2021, p. 1) describe Alzheimer's disease as an 'extreme case' of 'ambiguous loss' whereby 'the person is perceived as physically present but psychologically absent'. Johansson et al. (2013) compared dementia and cancer carers' experiences using the Anticipatory Grief Scale, noting that both groups began grieving their loved one's loss long before they died physically. While dementia's characteristics shape these outcomes, they are also profoundly socially shaped by how people frame dementia (Kevern, 2010; Kitwood, 1997; Sabat, 2008); there are relational, normative mechanisms operating in the allying of dementia, social death and anticipatory grief.

This allying has, however, been critiqued. For example, Brannelly (2011) demonstrates that when people living with dementia are considered socially dead, they are more likely to be disregarded, dehumanised and excluded. George (2010) argues that presuming anticipatory grief and social death take place creates a self-fulfilling prophecy, harming both carers and those cared for. He suggests challenging such presumptions, beginning with language, to generate a more helpful approach to ageing and dementia. Seeking to challenge these allegiances and alleviate their detrimental effects, yet nevertheless responding to the very real pain and grief associated with dementia, represents an aspirational balance, which might ultimately improve care for both people living with dementia and their carers.

Christianity is a diverse, complex religion, whose intersecting theologies of death, illness, suffering, personhood and care span many volumes. Certainly, though, Christianity acknowledges the painful realities of suffering, illness and death, sometimes (though not always) viewed as consequences of creation's fallen state (Hauerwas, 1986; Swinton, 2007; Hudson, 2016). Though relief is promised, this promise's complete fulfilment ultimately lies in the future; for now, Christians are offered a vision characterised by hope in the present and anticipation for the future. Christian theology also elevates humans' intrinsic value as created beings beloved to God (Genesis 1; Psalm 139). Moreover, many Christians emphasise the particular value of marginalised groups, considering them blessed and worthy of dignity, respect and full inclusion into the new vision of the world (Matthew 5:1–12).

Dementia has stimulated myriad theological responses. Drawing on lived experience, Post (2000; 2004) directly challenges suggestions that those living with dementia are 'already dead'. Swinton's work presents those living with dementia as precious to God and the church, and thus as spiritually alive (2017). Similarly, Friedrich, Woods and Williams (2021, p. 710) emphasise 'the continued presence of God in the lives of people living with dementia', but also acknowledge dementia's 'fundamental challenges' both theologically and experientially – not least for family and pastoral carers (p. 699). Kevern (2010) similarly describes dementia carers' 'soul-crushing, painful struggle against the departure of a loved one' (p. 238) as they become 'socially and politically invisible' (p. 243). Bons-Storm (2016) depicts fearfulness, hopelessness, loss and guilt, specifically naming dementia carers' 'false widow(er)hood' (pp. 1–4; see also Bryden, 2016; Mason, 2020). Hudson (2016, p. 51) presents dementia as a 'dreaded disease' through which people 'lose their personhood, or are in jeopardy of doing so', yet reasserts sufferers' human dignity as those created in the image of God (pp. 54–55).

Both in relation to dementia and more broadly, there is thus a balance to be struck in Christian theology between challenging anticipatory grief and social death, and recognising their often painful realities. Similarly, we have observed death studies scholarship dually framing dementia in terms of grief and challenging such approaches. This dual characterisation also underscores this chapter.

Method

The Educating for Inclusive, Caring Communities (EICC) project sought to develop non-problem-centred dementia teaching and training resources for prospective Christian ministers studying at UK Theological Education Institutes (TEIs) where few currently exist (Friedrich, Woods and Williams, 2021; Kevern, 2010). To inform the resources' design, we carried out semi-structured interviews with: people living with dementia and their carers (Mason, 2020); and staff at TEIs representing a range of Christian denominations (see Table 6.1) across the UK (see Table 6.2). We emailed TEI staff, inviting them to consider participating and/or

Table 6.1 Frequency of denominations of TEIs at which participants worked

Denomination	n
Anglican	6
Baptist	2
Church of Scotland	1
Free Church of Scotland	1
Methodist	1
Roman Catholic	2
United Reformed Church	1

68 J. Riley and J. Swinton

Table 6.2 Frequency of locations of TEIs at which participants worked

TEI location	n
England	10
Scotland	3
Northern Ireland	1

advertise the study at their organisation. The resulting sample included 15 individuals, representing 14 different TEIs (as some staff were employed at several institutions, and in some cases we interviewed more than one member of staff working at the same institution).

We approached Christian and secular dementia charities and specific churches, asking gatekeepers to share study details with people living with dementia and their carers. At the time of writing, the resulting sample included four people living with dementia and four carer-spouses. All eight had relationships with Christianity and one or more churches, but this was not a pre-requisite, and these relationships varied in character. We considered it important to directly hear the voices of people living with dementia (Hudson, 2016) and recognised that many dementia patients can provide informed consent. However, to safeguard those unable to consent, we restricted participation to those who retained legal and cognitive capacity, determined through conversations with gatekeepers, carers and the people living with dementia themselves. We did not need to exclude anybody on such bases; informed consent was given verbally or in writing in every case. The interviewer had training in conducting sensitive interviews with dementia patients. The University of Aberdeen Committee for Research Ethics and Governance in Arts, Social Sciences and Business granted ethical approval.

Interviews were conducted via video-conferencing, telephone or in-person (per interviewee preference) lasting 25–60 minutes, then transcribed, and coded using themes derived from the topic guides to aid comparison. We designed the interviews to be conversational, using topic guides flexibly and following interviewees' leads as to what was important. The topic guide for people living with dementia and their carers included: what it means to 'live well'; the relationship between faith and dementia; future hopes and fears; experiences seeking support from churches; and how churches might better support people living with dementia and their carers. The topic guide for theological educators included: theological questions and challenges associated with dementia; churches' role in, and capacity for, dementia care; and educational strategies for incorporating dementia in TEI curricula. Theological educators also shared personal and professional experiences of caring for people living with dementia in their congregations or families. As such, this chapter draws on data from both stakeholder groups, incorporating the voices of carers with diverse relationships to dementia and people living with it. All names are pseudonyms.

Findings

Dementia's grief, challenges and exclusion

Interviewees certainly depicted dementia's challenges and griefs. For example, Tabitha felt loss and sadness at her husband's illness:

> We've had a good life. We've done some great things and unfortunately [Ted] can't – this is a sadness – his memory's gone, so he can't remember a lot of the lovely things that we've done and that's – that's a shame. That's a huge loss actually.

While Ian felt well-supported by his local church, he nevertheless used 'respite', 'baggage' and 'problems' to describe carers' experiences, evoking difficulty:

> The [church group] is for both carers and the person with dementia. Trying to give the carers one hour's respite every Tuesday . . . because we're all together, we're all in the same boat. And we share our problems. It's a place where you can unload any baggage.

Ian and his wife Isobel also described their reactions to Isobel's diagnosis – reactions which directly anticipated death and evoked grief, including depression, shock, sadness, and composing a 'bucket list' (i.e., a list of things one wishes to do or experience before dying):

> When I was diagnosed, I went into a depression.. . . I didn't want to speak to anybody. I didn't want to go out. [Isobel]
> We went through all the crying processes of the shock of the dementia. And [Isobel] actually thought she was going to die very, very soon. So, what we decided to do is that we would make a bucket list. [Ian]

Elizabeth articulated the 'grief' of caring for someone with dementia most explicitly, saying:

> I think dementia is a different type of grieving. I think you're grieving while the person is still alive.

Carers also struggled when others excluded or avoided their loved ones on account of their dementia, contributing to a sense that their loved ones were socially dying, and evoking grief for their prior social livelihoods and identities. For example, it saddened Kate (whose mother lives with dementia) that people felt nervous and fearful, and thus avoided visiting her parents, isolating them socially:

> I think people are still, are nervous about going to visit [my parents]. . . There's always one or two who say, 'I'd love to visit. Do you think that would be OK?'. . . but then no one ever goes. And I think there's a fear in them of: what will they find?. . . how will they be able to talk to my Mam?

Rebecca associated this with broader social fear and 'taboo' surrounding ageing and dementia (see also Hudson, 2016):

I think it is a certain societal thing that we hate thinking about it . . . we're all a little bit terrified of dementia. So, we're far too scared to want to talk about it too much, and it feels a bit like a taboo subject.

Interviewees also identified this fear and resulting isolation within the church. For example, Sharon regularly drove her Mum and three other women (all of whom live with dementia) to coffee mornings at her church. She felt they were:

largely ignored by everybody!. . . they're just sat there on their own, nobody there is engaging with them. I think it's – there's a fear factor.

Ada, who has early-stage dementia, explained:

I get a lot of support from church.. . . They're aware. [But] I think they're frightened to get too close.

Melissa, who lives with dementia, recalled a conversation whereby:

The pastoral team was saying, 'Well, there's no point visiting XYZ because they've got dementia, they won't know whether you visited them or not'.

This presented people living with dementia as unable to benefit from or engage in reciprocal social interaction, and perpetuated further social isolation by denying them visits. Matthew described a man in his church congregation who:

sits next to his wife [in church] and it's rare for people to sit next to them. And she is always holding his hand, stopping him picking, pointing to the screen, helping him sit up. And I mean she must just be exhausted. Because you get a little picture of what she's doing for an hour on a Sunday of what she must be doing 24/7. . . she should be looking forward to coming to church because it's the one place that should be understood, where she feels that rest and help and care are available for her. And – and to the extent that he's able, he should be looking forward to church 'cause he feels like he belongs there.

Matthew characterised dementia care as challenging, resulting in 'exhaustion' and necessitating 'rest and help and care', and was concerned that this couple was ignored, and would feel they did not belong in the broader church fellowship whence such care might come. He also suggested that, typically:

Old age and dementia has to be one of the most significant spiritual battles people face at – and at exactly that stage of life church backs off and leaves you to your own devices.

'God hasn't given up on them' 71

Some interviewees had witnessed exclusion from churches' spiritual lives and worship, contributing to both spiritually and socially dying on account of their illness. For example, Matthew described some who believed that people living with dementia '[can't] benefit from the Bible teaching' at the heart of his evangelical church's worshipping life. While acknowledging that specific 'dementia-friendly' liturgy and services might be helpful in some cases, Geoff was one of several interviewees concerned that these implied people living with dementia were not welcome in other aspects of church worship:

> There are always going to be people in a congregation who are disturbed by people who 'disrupt' the service. I think that is sometimes why people with dementia are kind of separated.. . . I can understand why, maybe, you would have a service that is specifically aimed at folks with dementia, but I would much prefer if it's possible for those people to be included in the service and worship that everyone else is included in.

Several interviewees also highlighted the risk that losing the ability to travel to church independently might exacerbate social and spiritual isolation. Others had encountered more explicit exclusion. For example, Melissa described a church which:

> said – when they found out I had dementia, they said, 'Well, we don't want you coming here then'.

Tabitha recalled a gentleman with Alzheimer's who:

> used to sit on the end of the pew next to the aisle . . . and when people were queuing to go up for communion he put his walking stick out to trip them up. And eventually the vicar had to ask his wife not to bring him to church.

Resisting dementia as social or spiritual death

The above examples provide a snapshot of the grief and social and spiritual challenges experienced by carers and people living with dementia. But interviewees also resisted suggestions that dementia precipitated social and spiritual death. For example, Kate mused that:

> The church has often thought about ageing [as] synonymous with decay . . . as loss, as grief. As people not being able to do what they used to do.

However, she wanted to challenge this negative attitude. She reflected on Psalm 92:12–15 in this light:

> It said those who are ageing are, like, full of leaf and they're like green and leafy, and still – basically still bearing fruit . . .I think it's about setting the [church] culture . . . where it says that people with dementia are not a

72   *J. Riley and J. Swinton*

problem. That people with dementia, like any person, are a gift and a blessing and are to be treasured and loved and cared for . . .[and] seen as flourishing, as a leafy thing. And as a creation. And that God hasn't given up on them. And God is still working and then still shaping them, still forming them, still loving them, still growing them.

Others cited biblical accounts of God's heart for the disabled and unwell as grounds to challenge suggestions that people living with dementia could or should be viewed as spiritually or socially dead or dying. Catherine, for example, framed this in terms of being 'countercultural':

[It's about] the countercultural nature of [putting] at the centre of our church communities those who don't offer – you know, who aren't productive, aren't contributing in a capitalist, consumerist sense I think is what the Kingdom is about . . .[And] serving those who are in need, which is what we are about.

Being 'countercultural' by resisting dominant narratives and attitudes evident in society at large, and instead living according to God's 'Kingdom' values is a significant biblical theme (see John 15:18–19; John 17:14–16). For Catherine, being countercultural should see churches challenging 'capitalist, consumerist' ethoses which ascribe value in terms of contribution and production. Positioning being countercultural and caring for those in need as 'what we are about', Catherine evoked how she felt the church ('we') ought to care for people living with dementia, treating them as socially significant and valuable.

Some interviewees responded theologically to dementia by locating identity, permanence and security in God, not human memory or agency. For example, when Hannah's father had dementia before he died, she found it:

helpful to conceive of a person being held by God quite profoundly rather than the person needing to grasp onto God. [And someone I know had] a picture of God kind of cupping and holding my father in his hand and said, 'You know, God's got your dad, he's – he's not going anywhere for God'.

These are also important ideas in Swinton's seminal work on theology and dementia (2017, p. 257): 'Who am I?. . . the answer to that question lies in the hands of God, and I am at peace with that'.

Moreover, many interviewees had seen the benefits when individuals, communities and churches cared well for and valued people living with dementia. For example, while Elizabeth articulated the 'grief' she felt at her husband's illness, she was also grateful that going to church allowed him to continue being a 'very sociable person [who] likes people [and] enjoys talking to people'. Having cared for her father who had dementia before his death, Rebecca spoke positively about how his church community had helped him continue coming to church, and carry on hobbies integral to his identity and belonging:

In many ways his [Dad's] church did really well in that there were people who were aware of his condition [and] that he wanted to keep coming to church and that that familiarity was really important.. . . He was able to play the piano for half an hour before the toddler group met every Friday and that was a lovely thing.. . .[And] they made sure somebody came and picked him up [for church on Sundays].

Rebecca was one of several interviewees who emphasised familiarity, a theme observed by other researchers (e.g., Kennedy et al., 2014; Wrigley-Carr, 2021). She explained:

Liturgically, the familiarity was good [for Dad]. Singing was great, music for him was really key, and I mean even in his last months when I said the Lord's Prayer it was clear that he recognised it when he didn't recognise quite a lot of other things.

Like music and liturgy, others noted that personal prayer could create moments akin to paradoxical lucidity:

My father couldn't put a sentence together anymore, but when he and I would walk and pray together, he would start praying.. . . He couldn't talk anymore, but somehow the prayer words would come out. [Hannah]
My father had dementia and he still knew who God was. He didn't know who I was or didn't know where the bathroom was, and he could still pray to God and he could still talk about God even then. [Melissa]

Having seen her father's spiritual life continue in this way, Melissa felt hopeful for her own spiritual future amid dementia. She also shared several stories of friends living with dementia demonstrating ongoing spiritual vitality, setting these in sharp contrast to attitudes which reflected assumptions of spiritual and/or social death and dying among people living with dementia. She recalled one care nurse saying:

I don't know what you think [God's] got to do with you now and what it's got to do with your future.. . . How could you possibly know God still?

Because of such experiences, Melissa was determined that churches should:

believe that we can still be spiritually alive. That's so important because we are – the spiritual never dies, never dies.. . . And they need to be able to understand how to be more positive about it [dementia]. Because they think that when you get dementia, your faith dies. It does not die.

Melissa also described the importance of not excluding people living with dementia from actively serving the church by holding roles and responsibilities, describing these as 'something that they feel useful and valued by'. For Isobel, being able to hold such roles helped her feel 'part of the family', a sense of belonging which stands in sharp contrast to the experiences of social and spiritual exclusion explored above:

> [My husband] does readings in the church. And I'm on the rota for the door to welcome people into the church. So, we've got even, roles in the church. And you just feel part of the family.

Eleanor described one church which had, after some debate, come to recognise the importance of enabling people with dementia to hold roles, maintaining their belonging, and ensuring aspects of their spiritual and social identity could continue and thrive:

> There was a lovely lady who had quite early onset dementia. But she was part of the welcoming team . . .[and] used to help bringing people down from the altar steps back down into the nave [after communion]. And then she started to get more voluble, let's say. And there was an issue, because some people were coming back from communion and wanted to be quiet. And she was helping them down the steps but engaging in long conversations. And it took a kind of congregational meeting . . . to realise that that was [her] ministry. And if their silence had to be broken, well, actually it was a pretty small price to pay if she was still continuing that ministry . . . one or two took great offence.. . .[But] she was who she was and – and that had been her ministry up to then and – and why should it change?

Discussion

Interviewees articulated grief, social change and challenges associated with dementia, not least insofar as others' attitudes shaped their experiences. Equally, interviewees challenged and questioned how right or fair it was to frame those living with dementia as lost, socially insignificant, or spiritually or socially 'dead'. These two contrasting accounts echo two schools of thought evident within death studies scholarship: one which considers dementia an archetype of social death and associated anticipatory grief preceding physical death (Garand et al., 2012; Pérez-González et al., 2021; Johansson et al., 2013); and another which challenges these associations, arguing they cause harm (George, 2010; Brannelly, 2011). The evidence above suggests both schools can valuably illuminate Christian dementia carers' experiences, but only if taken together.

Christian theological responses have also both levelled theological challenges at cultural assumptions that people living with dementia undergo spiritual or social dying, and sought to acknowledge isolation, challenges, struggles and losses

(Friedrich, Woods and Williams, 2021; Kevern, 2010; Hudson, 2016). The account presented here certainly demands, with Bons-Storm (2016), that churches and theology must 'take this suffering seriously' (p. 6) and not 'deny the decisively great impact' dementia has on carers (p. 4). Yet they also require churches to echo Swinton's call to reorientate their theology such that people living with dementia and their carers might be remembered and included, and feel they belong, rather than excluded and treated as though already dead (2017).

In the spirit of practical theology, this chapter began with lived experience, and brought it into conversation with theological thinking and ideas (Mason, 2020). To fulfil the task of practical theology, we must next ask how Christian churches and communities might respond in practice to the dual dynamics at work in Christian dementia carers' experiences. This is particularly important in light of suggestions (Wrigley-Carr, 2021) that as cognitive abilities decline, religion's institutional elements take on especially weighty significance in maintaining people's spiritual identities. The findings above offer some practical insights. For example, churches might create rotas to provide transport to church for people living with dementia, and that they have opportunities to serve or share their gifts with others' support. This would help to safeguard their ongoing spiritual agency and social inclusion and facilitate the 'comfort and companionship' which Hudson (2016, p. 59) notes Christian worship can bestow upon people living with dementia and their carers, especially when it includes familiar rituals, music and prayer (Wrigley-Carr, 2021).

Equally, the same churches might host carers' groups, offering empathetic company, which can – as the above has shown – provide important support. Charitable initiatives such as Dementia Friendly Churches (Prama Foundation, 2019; Goodall and Hammond, n.d.) emphasise accessibility of church buildings and premises, and of service design. By critically evaluating and improving accessibility, churches could better ensure that people living with dementia can engage with services, with their specific, changed and changing needs accommodated. But, depending on particular needs, churches might also consider hosting designated accessible services, evaluating whether these might support the spiritual lives of people living with dementia, or risk sequestering them and their carers, risking greater social isolation, and at the expense of beneficial social connection and belonging.

Preaching might represent an opportunity to advocate the theological resistance explored above, inviting more members of a church fellowship to overcome fear and, in due course, to increase a congregation's capacity to include – rather than exclude – people living with dementia, and the impressions of social dying borne by their carers. As research by Epps et al. (2021a) has shown, intentionally addressing congregational attitudes can significantly transform perceptions of dementia, moving from negative towards more positive framings, which is important for both people living with dementia and their carers (Epps et al., 2021b). Yet the pulpit might also be a place to acknowledge the challenges and suffering illnesses such as dementia may create. Each of these possible responses requires careful consideration of how best to balance space for carers' grief and pain with narratives and responses that mitigate and counteract the social and spiritual change – even decline – that dementia can bring. It is also important to emphasise that this will

76 *J. Riley and J. Swinton*

require training and resources, and the building up of both clergy and laity (Friedrich, Woods and Williams, 2020). Churches may then become places 'of belonging, where people with dementia and those who offer care and support to them can find a place that is truly theirs and within which they can express the full experience of dementia – its pain, its affliction, and its lament as well as its joys and its possibilities' (Swinton, 2017, p. 278).

Indeed, the Judeo-Christian tradition of lament – 'a very particular form of prayer . . . that takes the brokenness of the human experience into the heart of God . . . an act of faithfulness in situations where faith and hope are challenged' (Swinton, 2007, p. 115) – both epitomises and actualises balance between grief and faithfulness, spiritual challenge and spiritual vitality. It represents one possible starting point for churches seeking to hear pain, but challenge elision between dementia, social death, and spiritual dying.

Conclusion

It has been suggested that dementia carers experience anticipatory grief, as both the disease trajectory and people's responses to it cause people living with dementia to undergo social death before they die physically. The qualitative data – concerning the experiences of people living with dementia, and of those who care for them in both pastoral and familial capacities - used in this chapter both support and counteract such suggestions. On the one hand, interviewees had certainly experienced the grief, challenges and losses dementia could bring, not least insofar as others treated people living with dementia differently, and – often – excluded them. On the other hand, they shared both personal experiences and theological rationales which encouraged them to resist suggestions that people living with dementia are socially or spiritually 'dead' or 'dying'. The sum of these somewhat contradictory experiences sees carers of people living with dementia needing support both in their grief and pain, and in their resistance. Interviewees' narratives also included examples of how churches might support both people living with dementia and their carers in ways which meets both needs, staunchly defending their spiritual and social inclusion while also offering support which acknowledges the challenges undoubtedly encountered.

References

Alzheimer's Society (2014) *Dementia UK Report*. London: Alzheimer's Society. Available at:www.alzheimers.org.uk/about-us/policy-and-influencing/dementia-uk-report(accessed 24 May 2023).

Bons-Storm, M. (2016) 'Where is God when dementia sneaks into our house? Practical theology and the partners of dementia patients', *HTS Theological Studies*, 72(4), p. a3227. Available at: https://doi.org/10.4102/hts.v72i4.3227.

Brannelly, T. (2011) 'Sustaining citizenship: People with dementia and the phenomenon of social death', *Nursing Ethics*, 18(5), pp. 662–671. Available at: https://doi.org/10.1177/0969733011408049.

Bryden, C. (2016) 'A spiritual journey into the I-Thou relationship: A personal reflection on living with dementia', *Journal of Religion, Spirituality and Aging*, 28(1–2), pp. 7–14. Available at: https://doi.org/10.1080/15528030.2015.1047294.

Cashin, Z. et al. (2019) 'Involving people with dementia and their carers in dementia education for undergraduate healthcare professionals: A qualitative study of motivation to participate and experience', *International Psychogeriatrics*, 31(6), pp. 869–876. Available at: https://doi.org/10.1017/S1041610218001357.

Collins, K.S. et al. (2007) 'Tending the soul: A teaching module for increasing student sensitivity to the spiritual needs of older adults', *Educational Gerontology*, 33(9), pp. 707–722. Available at: https://doi.org/10.1080/03601270701364420.

Davies, D.J. (2015) *Mors Britannica: Lifestyle and Death Style in Britain Today*. Oxford: Oxford University Press.

Davies, D.J. (2017) *Death, Ritual, and Belief: The Rhetoric of Funerary Rites*, 3rd edition. London: Oxford University Press.

Epps, F. et al. (2021a) 'Perceptions and attitudes toward dementia in predominantly African American congregants', *Journal of Applied Gerontology*, 40(11), pp. 1511–1516. Available at: https://doi.org/10.1177/0733464820987350.

Epps, F. et al. (2021b) 'A dementia-friendly church: How can the African American church support families affected by dementia?', *Dementia*, 20(2), pp. 556–569. Available at: https://doi.org/10.1177/1471301219900416.

Fahey-McCarthy, E. et al. (2009) 'Developing an education intervention for staff supporting persons with an intellectual disability and advanced dementia', *Journal of Policy and Practice in Intellectual Disabilities*, 6(4), pp. 267–275. Available at: https://doi.org/10.1111/j.1741-1130.2009.00231.x.

Farrow, M. et al. (2018) 'Improving knowledge and practice through massive open online dementia education: The understanding dementia and preventing dementia MOOCs', *Alzheimer's and Dementia*, 14(7,4), pp. P233–P233. Available at: https://doi.org/10.1016/j.jalz.2018.06.2368.

Friedrich, R., Woods, B. and Williams, S. (2021) "Just because the mind is confused it doesn't mean the spirit is confused': Exploring the role of Anglican clergy in ministry to persons with dementia', *Dementia*, 20(2), pp. 698–716. Available at: https://doi.org/10.1177/1471301220910572.

Garand, L. et al. (2012) 'Anticipatory grief in new family caregivers of persons with mild cognitive impairment and dementia', *Alzheimer Disease and Associated Disorders*, 26(2), pp. 159–165. Available at: https://doi.org/10.1097/WAD.0b013e31822f9051.

George, D.R. (2010) 'Overcoming the social death of dementia through language', *The Lancet*, 376(9741), pp. 586–587. Available at: https://doi.org/10.1016/S0140-6736(10)61286-X.

Goh, A.M. et al. (2022) 'Co-designing a dementia-specific education and training program for home care workers: The 'Promoting Independence Through Quality Dementia Care at Home' project', *Dementia*, 21(3), pp. 899–917. Available at: https://doi.org/10.1177/14713012211065377.

Goodall, M. and Hammond, G. (no date) 'Growing dementia-friendly churches: A practical guide'. Available at: www.mha.org.uk/files/3814/0931/8295/Growing_Dementia_Friendly_Churches.pdf (accessed 24 May 2023).

Gore, J. et al. (2022) 'A mixed-methods formative evaluation of a dementia-friendly congregation program for black churches', *International Journal of Environmental Research and Public Health*, 19(8), 4498. Available at: https://doi.org/10.3390/ijerph19084498.

Hauerwas, S. (1986) *Suffering Presence: Theological Reflections on Medicine, the Mentally Handicapped, and the Church*. Notre Dame, IN: University of Notre Dame Press.

Hudson, R.E. (2016) 'God's faithfulness and dementia: Christian theology in context', *Journal of Religion, Spirituality and Aging*, 28(1–2), pp. 50–67. Available at: https://doi.org/10.1080/15528030.2015.1041669.

Johansson, A.K. et al. (2013) 'Anticipatory grief among close relatives of persons with dementia in comparison with close relatives of patients with cancer', *The American Journal of Hospice and Palliative Care*, 30(1), pp. 29–34. Available at: https://doi.org/10.1177/1049909112439744.

Kennedy, E. et al. (2014) 'Christian worship leaders' attitudes and observations of people with dementia', *Dementia*, 13(5), pp. 586–597. Available at: https://doi.org/10.1177/1471301213479786.

Kevern, P. (2010) 'Alzheimer's and the dementia of God', *International Journal of Public Theology*, 4(2), pp. 237–253. Available at: https://doi.org/10.1163/156973210X491895.

Kevern, P. and Walker, M. (2013) 'Religious communities: What can they offer?', *Journal of Dementia Care*, 21, pp. 26–28.

Kitwood, T.M. (1997) *Dementia Reconsidered: The Person Comes First*. Milton Keynes: Open University Press.

Lindemann, E. (1963) 'Symptomatology and management of acute grief', *Pastoral Psychology*, 14, pp. 8–18. Available at: https://doi.org/10.1007/BF01770375.

Mason, J. (2020) 'Attending to the suffering of dementia: A practical theology approach', *Journal of Pastoral Theology*, 30(2), pp. 107–120. Available at: https://doi.org/10.1080/10649867.2019.1702794.

Moon, P.J. (2016) 'Anticipatory grief: A mere concept?', *American Journal of Hospice and Palliative Medicine*, 33(5), pp. 417–420. Available at: https://doi.org/10.1177/1049909115574262.

Pérez-González, A., Vilajoana-Celaya, J. and Guàrdia-Olmos, J. (2021) 'Alzheimer's disease caregiver characteristics and their relationship with anticipatory grief', *International Journal of Environmental Research and Public Health*, 18(16), pp. 8838. Available at: https://doi.org/10.3390/ijerph18168838.

Post, S.G. (2000) *The moral challenge of Alzheimer disease: Ethical issues from diagnosis to dying*. Baltimore, MD: JHU Press.

Post, S.G. (2004) 'Alzheimer's and grace', *First Things: A Monthly Journal of Religion and Public Life*, 142, pp. 12–15. Available at: www.firstthings.com/article/2004/04/alzheimers-grace (accessed 31 January 2024).

Powers, S. et al. (2020) 'Improving dementia capability among law enforcement: Evaluation of dementia education training in San Diego county', *Innovation in Aging*, 4(Supplement 1), p. 495. Available at: https://doi.org/10.1093/geroni/igaa057.1600.

Prama Foundation (2019) *Dementia friendly church resource pack*. Available at: https://dffw.org/wp-content/uploads/2021/03/Dementia-Friendly-Church.pdf (accessed 09 February 2024).

Sabat, S. (2008) 'A bio-psycho-social approach to dementia', in M. Downs and B. Bowers (eds) *Excellence in Dementia Care: Research into Practice*. Milton Keynes, UK: Open University Press, pp. 70–84.

Swinton, J. (2007) *Raging with Compassion: Pastoral Responses to the Problem of Evil*. Grand Rapids, MI: Eerdmans.

Swinton, J. (2017) *Dementia: Living in the Memories of God*, 2nd edition. London: SCM Press.

WHO (2024) *Dementia*. Geneva: World Health Organisation. Available at: www.who.int/health-topics/dementia (accessed 30 January 2024).

Wrigley-Carr, R. (2021) 'Corporate worship for people with dementia: Rituals and sensory stimulation', *Journal of Religion, Spirituality and Aging*, 33(2), pp. 206–222. Available at: https://doi.org/10.1080/15528030.2020.1837332.

7 The grief of care partners of people living and dying with dementia

A psychodynamic perspective

Phil McEvoy, Esther Ramsay-Jones, Amanda Barrell, Rachel Yates-Hoyles and Emma Smith

Introduction

Dementia is an umbrella term for a diverse range of life-limiting neurocognitive disorders, which progressively affect people's memory, cognitive reasoning skills, ability to communicate, physical health, and capacity to care for themselves (Sachdev et al., 2014). Alzheimer's disease and other forms of dementia are now the leading cause of death in England and Wales (Office for National Statistics, 2023). Efforts have been made to improve service provision for people with dementia and their relatives (Department of Health, 2009), but relatively little space has been given to the notion of dying well with dementia. The death of people with dementia involves fundamental changes in their relationship with their care partners whom they rely on for assistance and support. The shift towards increasing dependency can generate powerful internal conflicts that can affect their care partner's ability to mourn and adapt to their changing circumstances.

This chapter examines the grief of care partners of people with dementia from a psychodynamic perspective. It focuses on four aspects of the grief associated with living and dying with dementia: anticipatory grief, ambiguous loss, disenfranchised grief and dying with dementia. The testimonies of care partners, who have been supported by Age UK Salford, shed light on the complexity of their grief and the emotional challenges they face.

Psychodynamic perspective on grief

Grief is a biologically triggered emotional response to the separation and distress people feel following a significant loss (Panksepp and Watt, 2011). Viewed through a psychodynamic lens, the sadness, confusion, and pining people feel when they are grieving can be viewed as the price they pay for their love and attachments (Parkes and Prigerson, 2013). Mourning is an adaptive response to grief that normally eases over time, as they come to terms with the reality of their loss. However, grief can take an alternative form as it becomes frozen in a state of melancholia (Freud, 1917). This is a complex and particularly painful form of grief that manifests itself in inner emptiness, despondency, and the drain of energy for living that is fuelled by confusion about the nature of the loss and attacks upon the self (Agass,

DOI: 10.4324/9781003435365-7

80   *P. McEvoy et al.*

2013). The capacity to live with uncertainties may be severely curtailed as people who are experiencing intense, melancholic grief feel abandoned by others who do not understand their loss (Klein, 1946). The distinctions between grief, mourning and melancholia, are not trivial, but often unclear. To varying degrees, those who are grieving carry them within the different parts of themselves. To an attuned listening ear, this dynamic may be ever-present, but it is often hidden behind a mask of putting on a brave face to the world.

Partners of people living and dying with dementia

Care partners play a vital role in enabling people with dementia to sustain their independence and quality of life by providing practical assistance, emotional support, and liaising with formal health and social care services on their behalf. The impact of caregiving varies; for some, being a care partner can be a valued experience, but it is also an exhausting and demanding one. Due to the gendered nature of much unpaid and paid care work, this is a responsibility that is disproportionately shouldered by women (Mielke, Vemuri and Rocca, 2014).

As dementia advances, aspects of their partner's changed behaviour, such as repetitively asking the same questions, can sometimes feel unbearable to deal with. Care partners often feel an acute sense of loss for the person they knew and find it difficult to accept the changes in their relationship (Moore et al., 2023). They are at increased risk of depression and anxiety-related mental health problems (Abreu et al., 2020), which are linked to these stresses, and at high risk of developing a prolonged and complicated grief reaction. The prevalence of complicated grief in bereaved partners is estimated to be between 10% and 20% (Shear, 2010). Depending upon the type of dementia, their personality, the circumstances in which they live, and the stage of the dementia trajectory, individual care partners may be affected in differing ways (Egilstrod, Rayn and Petersen, 2019). However, common factors that may add to the complexity of the grieving process for the care partners of people with dementia include

i. anticipatory grief,
ii. ambiguous loss,
iii. disenfranchised grief and
iv. dying with dementia.

Anticipatory grief

Anticipatory grief is a response to impending loss that may be equivalent in its intensity and duration to the grief of the bereaved following a death (Meuser and Marwit, 2001). For care partners of people living with dementia, these losses can include the difficulty in laying down new memories experienced by their partner, limitations in their ability to communicate, as well as the loss of a feeling of reciprocity in their relationship and their ability to connect through their shared history

The grief of care partners 81

(Garner, 1997). The care partners' anticipatory grief may be particularly intense at transition points in the dementia journey, such as receiving a diagnosis, increased care needs, communication changes, moving into a care home and the anticipated death of their partners.

The meaning the care partner attaches to their partner's increasing vulnerability and loss of independence may be connected to the social context and the dynamic of their familial relationships. The psychotherapist and researcher Sandra Evans (2020) cites an example of Mark (a son) and Jools (his mother), an ex-nurse diagnosed with Alzheimer's in her mid-eighties. Their close bond was reinforced, Jools was able to utilise her retained knowledge in tandem with Mark's more agile mind and problem-solving abilities. Together, they found new ways of coping as Jools became increasingly muddled. However, relationships are rarely so straightforward. As care partners anticipate the suffering that lies in store for the person with dementia, they have to find a balance between attending to their own needs and making sacrifices in order to support their partner. It is common for carers to be racked with guilt as they can feel 'selfish' as they make difficult choices and live with worries about the future. Young care partners, in particular, may pine for landmark events that they will miss out on. The envy they feel when they foresee their peers having opportunities that they will be denied can evoke feelings of shame that are especially hard to deal with (Hall and Sikes, 2017). Anxieties triggered by anticipatory grief are likely to be most heavily defended against when they resonate with relational conflicts and previous losses that have not been mourned. For example, in the biographical film Iris, the anticipatory grief of John, the husband of the philosopher and novelist Iris Murdoch, came to the fore at the funeral of Janet, one of their best friends. When John encountered one of Iris's ex-lovers Maurice, his unconscious resentments and guilt that had been suppressed were laid bare. John vented his fury towards Iris, as he contemplated having to arrange for her to be admitted to a care home (Anderson, 2010).

For practitioners who are supporting the partner of someone living with dementia, it is important to approach these anticipated losses with tact and sensitivity as to the timing of when best to broach them. It may not be easy to strike a balance between impinging upon their anticipated losses in too direct a way and being too detached, thereby conveying that their anticipated grief is too hard to talk about. It is important to be able to hold on to the anxieties, whilst simultaneously creating a containing space for thinking about their meaning and implications. Winnicott focussed on the necessity of patiently bearing with persecutory anxieties until carers can name them for themselves and move towards less heavily defended states of mind (Winnicott et al., 1989).

Ambiguous loss

An ambiguous loss is an experience of loss that resists closure due to the paradox of absence and presence (Boss, 1999). It is a liminal experience, one that has an 'as if' quality. It is difficult to locate and understand because it transgresses the emotional need we have for object constancy. Object constancy is the emotional drive we have to hold on to a stable representation in our mind, of the significance of the other to whom we are attached (Akhtar, 1994). Two different realities may have to be held in mind at the same time. The person with dementia is both the same person and not the person they once were. For their care partners, this is a disturbing experience to wrestle with and can arouse considerable emotional dissonance.

The anthropologist, Janelle Taylor (2008, p. 326) gave a moving account of her experience of ambiguous loss, as she mourned for the loss of her mother's mind and the relationship they once had:

> My mother would certainly fail a pop quiz about my name, but she lights up when she sees me. She is eager to talk, and tries to speak, but words often elude her, and sentences get distracted and wander off in unanticipated directions.

Taylor's experience was bitter-sweet. At an unconscious level, the lack of recognition and rejection she felt stirred up paranoid feelings towards her mother, which were difficult to accept. Yet, these moments of connection also helped her to sustain her deep love for her mother, which was reciprocated until the end of her life.

The losses of the carer and cared for in a relationship are very much intertwined, with each potentially affecting the other (Wray and Bergstrom, 2023). The care partner may feel lost as they question their identity and lose hold of their established sense of self, as their relationship to their partner becomes increasingly asymmetrical.

As the capacity to understand and hold on to their contradictory experiences of the person with dementia and of themselves becomes increasingly strained, it is common for care partners to slip into split states of mind in which the extent to which the person with dementia has changed is minimised or maximised. This tendency is reflected in tropes such as 'I deal with the person, not the dementia' and 'they are no longer the person they once were'.

Ambiguous loss can be very painful to accept, but the grief that is associated with this loss can be contained by engaging with the confusion that it generates, whilst maintaining an empathic stance towards the impact of 'not knowing'. There is a perceived wisdom that the internal world of people with dementia is infused with absence, which is impossible to make sense of (Basting, 2003). Yet, how things seem on the surface does not always reflect the picture that can be grasped when a situation can be engaged with and reflected upon. For example, in her recent book, *Travellers to unimaginable lands*, Dasha Kiper (2023) has highlighted how people with dementia fight to preserve their sense of self in meaningful ways.

A common response to changes in the relationship, is for the care partner to disengage or act out unarticulated frustrations, as they express their fear of losing control (Balfour, 2020). It is important for practitioners to acknowledge the inherent precariousness and uncertainty of the care partner's situation (Caleb, 2019), whilst tentatively drawing attention to the background thoughts they are having about their uncertainties and perceived losses, which may reflect their conflicting goals and internal stresses (McEvoy et al., 2013).

The grief of care partners 83

Disenfranchised grief

Disenfranchised grief is a stigmatised form of grief that cannot be publicly acknowledged due to the social taboos that surround the grief (Doka, 1999). In Western societies, which place a premium on independence, self-sufficiency and personal freedom, this grief is connected to the fear of losing one's mind and being dependent on others. The loss of independence is seen as a source of shame (Brown, 2020) as it exposes personal limitations and foregrounds questions about what it means to be vulnerable. Care partners often experience contradictory feelings that can be difficult to identify or talk about. On the one hand they can feel helpless as they are unable to prevent the cognitive decline and suffering of their partner with dementia, whilst on the other hand they feel guilty for harbouring feelings of anger that are triggered by the frustrations and strain of caregiving (Moore et al., 2023).

The grief experienced by those that are affected by dementia is widespread, but it is also hidden from view. It is contained in the segregated spaces of hospitals and care homes, or by social withdrawal from engagement with the wider community (Ramsay-Jones, 2019). Kiper highlights that 'the sad truth is that most caregivers end up feeling alone' (Kiper, 2023, p. 96). Internalised forms of disenfranchised grief can lead many care partners to minimise their emotional pain. They are careful not to burden others with their distress and say others have it a lot worse than they do.

In a poem from her collection *The Solitary*, Vuyelwa Carlin (2009, p. 39) describes the death of Hatty (1903–2003) in a care home:

Time to die: for two weeks
you ate nothing, drank nothing.
Dead, you were a bluish wisp –
malleable, miniature arms in lacy sleeves:
at last, we could fasten the fiddly pearl buttons,
brush out, dispose, your gorgeous, heavy, slaty, hair.

There is an absence of a relational field surrounding Hatty's death which mirrors the isolation that people with dementia can often experience (Kitwood, 1997). Perhaps we all share a collective sense of guilt and pay a social cost for dementia whose losses and deaths are rendered invisible (Lawton and Nahemow, 1973).

For practitioners working with care partners, it is also important to examine their own disenfranchised grief as they engage in the difficult work of bearing witness to those bereaved by dementia. All too often, the impact of their emotional labour is ignored, and practitioners are not well cared for themselves (Ramsay-Jones, 2020). The work they do has an inherent potential to reactivate their own losses and stir up feelings of shame. Their unexamined countertransference (Hinshelwood, 1999) can lead to emotional burn-out or the unintentional acting out of their personal issues in their work. Robust supervision and governance strategies and, in some cases, personal therapy may be necessary to examine their vicarious grief.

84 *P. McEvoy et al.*

Dying with dementia

Dementia-related disabilities accumulate until a state of absolute dependency is reached in the later stages of dementia. The life expectancy for people diagnosed with Alzheimer's disease can be up to 20 years (Tom et al., 2015). For much of this time, care partners often provide very high levels of assistance, while adjusting to the changes in the relationship as their spouse or parent with dementia experiences neurological decline. It is common for full-time care partners of people with moderate to severe dementia to become exhausted by the practical and emotional demands of caring. Sources of significant stress include agitation and aggressive questioning, pacing, sleep disturbance, the need for assistance with eating and drinking, and incontinence (Feast et al., 2016), plus diagnostic-specific symptoms such as visual hallucinations and movement disorders in dementia with Lewy Bodies. The direct and indirect financial impacts of being a dementia care partner are considerable and are disproportionately borne by those with the least ability to pay (Samuel et al., 2020), as are the emotional costs of caring for those that are the most isolated (Carbone et al., 2021). Being a care partner for someone with dementia strains family relationships and, in some families, this may be beyond breaking point (Lewis et al., 2014).

These stresses tend to intersect with ethnic and sociocultural variables, but they may ease if a partner is admitted to a care home, as the demands of providing one-to-one care are reduced. However, many care partners continue to have high levels of involvement as they advocate for the person with dementia, provide emotional support and offer practical assistance in the care home setting (Gaugler and Mitchell, 2022). Care partners can feel weighed down by guilt, owing to a sense of having abandoned their parent or spouse, in the face of their inevitable decline and death. As they move towards the end of life, this guilt is frequently aggravated by confusion over end-of-life decisions. In the absence of clear advance directives, it can be hard to be certain that end-of-life decisions are respectful of the personhood and wishes of partners with dementia who no longer have the capacity to consent (Sellars et al., 2019). The end of life can be sudden; it is common for people with dementia to die quickly with a chest infection or following a fall. The absence of an opportunity to say goodbye and have a shared conversation that may lend a sense of meaning and bring comfort can be traumatic, as it can add to the sense of moral injury (Shay, 2014) that carers carry about their failings.

Following the death of their significant other, care partners can experience anxieties, which may mirror the loss of the sense of self and relationship with others experienced by many people with dementia. The sense of existential crisis may be especially strong for carers who experience a sense of redundancy after their partner has died. Their life may feel empty without their relationship and caring responsibilities. Looking back retrospectively on the losses and isolation that have been an inherent aspect of their caregiving role can be frightening and emotionally painful. When they have been immersed with the day to day demands of caring, they may never have mourned for what this has actually meant (Nathanson and Rogers, 2020).

The grief of care partners 85

For practitioners, the suppressed anger that they may absorb in the transference from care partners they work with can be challenging to deal with. Having a model of grief to hold on to may help them to identify where their anger is coming from. The dementia grief model developed by Blandin and Pepin (2017) identifies the challenges which care partners may have in acknowledging the reality of their loss, tolerating difficult feelings, and adapting to their new life circumstances. Malan's (1976) two triangles approach may also be useful to help formulate a psychodynamic understanding of the care partner's response. The triangle of conflict represents the dominant impulse or feeling state, the anxiety, and the emotional defence of the care partner. The triangle of person represents their relationship with themselves, the deceased partner with dementia, and the practitioner.

Testimonies of care partners

The testimonies below come from bereaved dementia care partners who have attended the Empowered Conversations course and Empowered Carers sessions run by Age UK, Salford. The Empowered Conversations course is based on a model of practice called the Communication Empowerment Framework (Morris et al., 2020), which encourages carers to pay attention to the pragmatic features of their communicative interaction. A feasibility study (Morris et al., 2021) has shown that attending the course is associated with improvements in perceived stress and quality of communication that are sustained after the course has been completed. Empowered Carers sessions are designed to bolster the psychological resources of family carers of people with dementia, if they require more proactive emotional support. It is modelled on the structured approach to caregiver resilience-building pioneered by the New York University Caregiver Intervention (NYUCI) (Mittelman et al., 2004). Emotional support is provided by dementia practitioners with a counselling or mentoring background. It is designed to be open-ended, without any arbitrary time limit, although the frequency of the sessions may be titrated, ranging from weekly to monthly, depending on the needs of the care partners.

Interview methodology

Semi-structured interviews of approximately 30 minutes duration were conducted with five dementia care partners by the practitioners (AB and RYH) who have worked with them as part of an evaluative research project. The interviewees were purposefully selected because of their differing circumstances and experiences of loss. The interviews were conducted via Zoom and centred on the open-ended question of how loss had featured in their emotional journey. The interviewees gave their written consent to have the interviews filmed, recorded and analysed in order to gain an understanding of the grieving process experienced by care partners of people with a dementia, with the ethical approval of the Age UK steering group that oversees the Empowered Conversations and Empowered Carers projects. All the participants were aware that material from the interviews may also be used for dissemination and publication purposes. Transcripts of the interviews were brought

86 *P. McEvoy et al.*

to a reflective practice group (Balint, 1955; Bradley and Rustin, 2018), which was facilitated by an external practitioner-researcher (ERJ). A reflexive understanding of the care partners' testimonies was developed through group discussion and the technique of free association (Holmes, 2018). The quotes presented below have been preserved to maintain their authenticity but identifying information has been removed to preserve the care partner's confidentiality. All the carers interviewed were White British. Four of the carers had cared for one of their parents and one for her husband. Three of the interviewees were female and two were male.

Interview findings

Driven by their love, commitment, and perhaps more complex elements of attachment bonds, often difficult to acknowledge, all the carers had provided very high levels of care for their spouse or parent as they lived and died with dementia. Their responses to the question of how loss featured in their emotional journey were infused with humility. There was a tone of understatement, when they talked about the personal sacrifices they had made, at great personal cost, which is captured in the following reflection of a care partner (Interviewee 1), who had cared for her husband, of over 50 years, in the last years of his life:

> He wasn't the person I knew. We'd been together for a long time. He changed in subtle ways. He gradually withdrew and wasn't the person I married. It was quite difficult to cope with that. Looking back, he didn't realise what was happening. He thought that he was still the same. That's hard in terms of loss because you've still got to carry on doing what you've got to do.

Some of the interviews were painful to watch, as some of the care partners wrestled with traumatic aspects of their loss, whereas others seemed to be more at peace. However, the care partners conveyed a sense of appreciation that their loss was recognised and understood, by a practitioner who had accompanied them for a substantial part of their emotional journey. The elements of anticipatory grief, ambiguous loss, and disenfranchised grief, highlighted in the discussion above, were present – with some nuances.

Anticipatory grief

For some of the care partners, the experience of anticipatory grief was immediate and stark. Dementia was experienced by the care partner (Interviewee 3) quoted below as a 'sledgehammer' that threatened to destroy his relationship with his mother and sense of self:

> At the very, very beginning of the process of identifying and realising that my mother had dementia I felt a very profound sense of loss. I think it hit me quite out of the blue in a way because I had this wonderful relationship with my mother that . . . I could, I could sense that this would be taken away from me. Things slipping away, moving in a direction that I didn't want it to go.

The grief of care partners   87

For this care partner, the ability to acknowledge what was happening was linked to previous discussions he had with his mum and family in which they had clarified his mum's prior wishes. The sense of anticipatory grief was much cloudier for other care partners, who experienced it as a gradual dawning that their hopes for their future were being foreclosed. The question of 'Do I want to know more about this?' was hard to engage with because it amplified their fears, as did a lack of clarity over the precise diagnosis, or an understanding of what the implications of the diagnosis would be. This sense of confusion was exemplified by a care partner (Interviewee 1) whose husband had dementia with Lewy Bodies:

> I don't think you could prepare yourself because it really is the unknown. You read about dementia. There's so many different forms of dementia. I think the difficulty is that it's all lumped into one umbrella.

Ambiguous loss

In the earlier stages of their dementia, the care partners' ambiguous loss was experienced as confusing and frustrating. It was hard to accept the uncharacteristic changes, as a person – mother, father, spouse – became fractious, or withdrawn. Yet, as the trajectory of the dementia progressed, the care partners responded to this ambiguous loss in differing ways. Some of the care partners held on to the ambiguity as a resource. They looked forward to the rare moments of lucidity and connection. These moments became a source of comfort that helped them to accept their partners for who they now were. This was especially the case in the later stages of dementia when the tangles of dementia released their suffocating grip, all too briefly. The sustaining power of these rare moments was captured in the words of a daughter (Interviewee 2) who described how her dad, who had lost the ability to maintain verbal conversation, could sometimes speak through his eyes:

> For him to look so blank when you're having a conversation, that was hard. You didn't know whether he was understanding what you're saying or not. That was hard, but then just out of the blue he'd get his little twinkle in his eye, and it was like his mischief look and we'd get a smile. And you know what, those moments were so amazing and we both . . . we both embraced them.

Other care partners found this ambiguity harder to accept. One of the care partners (Interviewee 4) described the ambiguous loss as a threat. It brought back difficulties in his relationship with his mother that he would have preferred to relinquish. He could accept his mum as she was before her dementia and later when she was in the end-of-life stage, but the ambiguities of the fluctuations in between, aroused feelings of paranoia. Emotionally exhausted by a catalogue of adversities and losses, he likened his experience to that of being stuck in an emotional black hole:

> In some ways the whole process was sort of steeped in loss, my father died and literally six months on from my father dying my mum got dementia, well

88   *P. McEvoy et al.*

she got the memory dimension. I still feel now, three to four years later, that I've not had time to process any of that. The whole experience of caring for my mum was cast in that kind of foundry of loss. It was horrible.

Disenfranchised grief

The sense of alienation which some of the care partners harboured could be seen as a form of disenfranchised grief that was located in their internal state of mind, as well as their social circumstances. A daughter (Interviewee 5) who was a full-time carer for her mum, who had severe dementia and was living at home, lost contact with friends and family. In her interview, it was clear that she was battling to recover lost parts of herself after what had been an all-consuming and isolating experience. She recounted that even when her family came to see her, she was often left in a position in which she had to reorder her priorities and break off from talking to them, to attend to her mum's needs:

> Sometimes it feels like you've lost yourself, because you are that busy and intent in looking after somebody. And finding yourself afterwards, I've still not done it . . . . When you've been looking after someone like that, it really does take over your life.

Elements of this loss of self-identity were also apparent when the care partners spoke about the impact of the decision they had reluctantly made to transfer their spouse or parent to a care home. When they no longer had the resources to care for them at home, it felt like a betrayal of their spousal or filial responsibility. This relinquishing of their ego ideal (Freud, 1923) left them feeling depleted, as they no longer saw themselves as the person they were before. Their sense of personal devastation was exemplified by a daughter (Interviewee 2) who spoke about how her dad was admitted to a care home during the time when strict COVID regulations were in place that prevented relatives from visiting:

> When dad went into the home and . . . um . . . I mean it was difficult because they had COVID and we couldn't go in for a month and that was heartbreaking because I'd gone a month already, with him being in hospital and I couldn't see him and that was really, really hard.

Disenfranchised grief is often discussed at a societal level, but it was clear from the interviews that this is a complex construct that involves psychic components. Care partners withdrew from interaction with others to shield themselves from further demands upon their time and resources that they did not have the emotional capacity to cope with. One of the care partners (Interviewee 5) spoke about the boundaries that she had to put in place to protect herself, as she felt increasingly overwhelmed:

> It makes it worse because other people still expect you to be at their beck and call . . . to do what they want you to do and sometimes you don't want to be bothered. They say just give me a call, but you may not want to talk to them.

The grief of care partners   89

This sense of disenfranchisement was also resisted by some of the care partners in other ways. For example, contra to the pull towards disenfranchisement there was a quality of acceptance, derived from the finding of meaning and renewed strength, that resonated with the generative response to loss identified by writers such as David Kessler (2019) and Victor Frankl (2006). A poignant example of this sense-making was provided by a care partner (Interviewee 3) who shared a story about the mutual gratitude that he and his mum had for the life they had shared together:

And I put her into bed and I'd say good night and then she'd say to me . . . she'd look me in the eye and she'd say 'well thank you for everything' and I would just think wow you know that is a direct comment to me. Um . . . and it encompassed so much you know. It's . . . it's a very short sentence but it's loaded with meaning because and I . . . I needed that at the end of every day.

Summary of findings

Four points stood out from the interviews.

First, anticipatory grief is a form of grief that is intermingled with fears about the future. The anticipatory grief of the care partners was linked to the clarity of understanding regarding the implications of a diagnosis of different types of dementia, as well as the care partner's emotional resources and relationship with their partner.

Second, the uncertainty surrounding their ambiguous loss was experienced in many ways. Ambiguous loss may be a source of confusion, a means of holding on to a secure attachment to a partner, or a reminder of prior experiences that care partners of people with dementia may consciously or unconsciously want to disavow.

Third, disenfranchised grief is a complex construct, with layers of meanings that are influenced by the societal stigma that still surrounds dementia and the care partners' internal response to their losses. The disenfranchised grief of some of the care partners was embroiled with internalised feelings of guilt, but other care partners resisted their disenfranchised grief and gave themselves permission to mourn.

Fourth, the accumulated loss and traumas that care partners of people with dementia experience, both before and after the death of their partner, can be severely depleting and have a profound impact on their sense of self. Some of the care partners interviewed felt extremely isolated and abandoned in their grief. Breakdowns in the felt sense of connection with their partner were especially difficult to bear when they affected the care partners' ability to connect with the sustaining aspects of their relationships.

Conclusion

In common with previous psychodynamic works on the experiences of family carers of people who are living and dying of dementia (Davenhill, 2007; Dartington, 2006; Ramsay-Jones, 2019; Evans, Garner and Darnley-Smith, 2020), this chapter has highlighted the importance of continuity in the relational field. The concepts of anticipatory grief, ambiguous loss, disfranchised grief and accumulated loss shed

90   P. McEvoy et al.

light on the dynamics of the relational context. They illustrate the many layers of complexity that contribute to the carers' yearnings and the emotional challenges that can affect their ability to mourn their losses. For example, their fears about the future, their response to uncertainty, differences in giving themselves permission to mourn and, for some, a sense of isolation and abandonment. All the care partners experienced acute emotional pain that stemmed from their relational loss, but there were clear differences in the interviewee's trajectories of grief as they responded to these losses in different, sometimes fluctuating, ways.

The interviewees benefited from having access to containing emotional spaces (Bion, 1962) in which they could talk about their losses, fears, guilt and regrets. While family, friends or communal groups may provide vital support to carers, it may not be easy for care partners to talk to them about the depth of their feelings and the impact of their loss on their sense of self. This points to the need for more professional counselling support to help care partners to deal with acute pre-death grief and for bereaved carers who are emotionally exhausted following the death of their partner.

A limitation of the evaluative research project was that the interviewees came from a relatively homogenous white British social group and there were not enough interviews conducted to differentiate between the grief experiences of care partners from different social groups. It is important to bear in mind that the experiences of young care partners, working care partners with multiple responsibilities, so called 'sandwich' carers and older spouses who care for their life partners may be very different. It may be necessary to examine the emotional journeys of care partners from differing ethnicities and cultural locales to gain a better understanding of the socio-cultural aspects of their experiences of grief. Evidence suggests that care partners who are from ethnic and sexual minority groups may feel particularly unsupported (Nolan, Kirkland and Davis, 2021).

References

Abreu, W. et al. (2020) 'A cross-sectional study of family caregiver burden and psychological distress linked to frailty and functional dependency of a relative with advanced dementia', *Dementia*, 19(2), pp. 301–318. Available at: https://doi.org/10.1177/1471301218773842.

Agass, R. (2013) 'Clinical reflections on self-attack', *Psychoanalytic Psychotherapy*, 27(3), pp. 228–247. Available at: https://doi.org/10.1080/02668734.2013.829117.

Akhtar, S. (1994) 'Object constancy and adult psychopathology', *The International Journal of Psychoanalysis*, 75(3), pp. 441–455.

Anderson, D. (2010) 'Love and hate in dementia: The depressive position in the film Iris', *The International Journal of Psychoanalysis*, 91(5), pp. 1289–1297. Available at: https://doi.org/10.1111/j.1745-8315.2010.00324.x.

Balfour, A. (2020) 'The fragile thread of connection', in S. Evans, J. Garner and R. Darnley-Smith (eds) *Psychodynamic Approaches to the Experience of Dementia: Perspectives from Observation, Theory and Practice*. London: Routledge, pp. 118–132.

Balint, M. (1955) 'The doctor, his patient, and the illness', *The Lancet*, 265(6866), pp. 683–688. Available at: https://doi.org/10.1016/S0140-6736(55)91061-8.

Basting, A.D. (2003) 'Looking back from loss: Views of the self in Alzheimer's disease', *Journal of Aging Studies*, 17(1), pp. 87–99. Available at: https://doi.org/10.1016/S0890-4065(02)00092-0.

The grief of care partners 91

Bion, W.R. (1962) *Learning from Experience*. London: Heinemann.

Blandin, K. and Pepin, R. (2017) 'Dementia grief: A theoretical model of a unique grief experience', *Dementia*, 16(1), pp. 67–78. Available at: https://doi.org/10.1177/147130121 5581081.

Boss, P. (1999) *Ambiguous Loss*. Cambridge, MA: Harvard University Press.

Bradley, J. and Rustin, M. (2018) *Work Discussion: Learning from Reflective Practice in Work with Children and Families*. London: Routledge.

Brown, J. 2020 'Prognosis and planning: Advanced care planning through a psychoanalytic frame', in S. Evans, J. Garner and R. Darnley-Smith (eds) *Psychodynamic Approaches to the Experience of Dementia: Perspectives from Observation, Theory and Practice*. London: Routledge, pp. 41–55.

Caleb, A.M. (2019) 'Embracing the negative capability of dementia', *Survive and Thrive: A Journal for Medical Humanities and Narrative as Medicine*, 4(1), 12. Available at: https://repository.stcloudstate.edu/survive_thrive/vol4/iss1/12/ (accessed 31 January 2024).

Carbone, E.A. et al. (2021) 'The mental health of caregivers and their patients with dementia during the COVID-19 pandemic: A systematic review', *Frontiers in Psychology*, 12, 6070. Available at: https://doi.org/10.3389/fpsyg.2021.782833.

Carlin, V. (2009) *The Solitary*. Bridgend: Seren.

Dartington, T. (2006) 'Managing vulnerability', *Dementia*, 5(4), pp. 475–478. Available at: https://doi.org/10.1177/1471301206069901.

Davenhill, R. (2007) *Looking into Later Life: A Psychoanalytic Approach to Depression and Dementia in Old Age*. London: Karnac Books.

Department of Health (2009). *Living Well with Dementia: A National Dementia Strategy*. London: Department of Health. Available at: https://assets.publishing.service.gov.uk/media/5a7a15a7ed915d6eaf153a36/dh_094051.pdf (accessed 2 February 2024).

Doka, K.J. (1999) 'Disenfranchised grief', *Bereavement Care*, 18(3), pp. 37–39. Available at: https://doi.org/10.1080/02682629908657467.

Egilstrod, B., Ravn, M.B. and Petersen, K.S. (2019) 'Living with a partner with dementia: A systematic review and thematic synthesis of spouses' lived experiences of changes in their everyday lives', *Aging and Mental Health*, 23(5), pp.541–550. Available at: https://doi.org/10.1080/13607863.2018.1433634.

Evans, S. (2020) 'The experience of loss in dementia: Melancholia without the mourning?', in S. Evans, J. Garner and R. Darnley-Smith (eds) *Psychodynamic Approaches to the Experience of Dementia: Perspectives from Observation, Theory and Practice*. London: Routledge, pp. 56–68.

Evans, S., Garner, J. and Darnley-Smith, R. (2020) *Psychodynamic Approaches to the Experience of Dementia: Perspectives from Observation, Theory and Practice*. London: Routledge.

Feast, A. et al. (2016) 'Behavioural and psychological symptoms in dementia and the challenges for family carers: Systematic review', *The British Journal of Psychiatry*, 208(5), pp. 429–434. Available at: https://doi.org/10.1192/bjp.bp.114.153684.

Frankl, V.E. (2006) *Man's Search for Meaning*. London: Rider.

Freud, S. (1917) 'Mourning and melancholia', in J. Strachey, (ed.) *The Standard Edition of the Complete Psychological Works of Sigmund Freud*. London: Hogarth Press, Volume 14, pp. 237–258.

Freud, S. (1923) 'The Ego and the Id', in J. Strachey (ed.) *The Standard Edition of the Complete Psychological works of Sigmund Freud*. London: Hogarth Press, Volume 19, pp. 1–59.

Garner, J. (1997) 'Dementia: An intimate death', *British Journal of Medical Psychology*, 70, pp. 177–184. Available at: https://doi.org/10.1111/j.2044-8341.1997.tb01897.x.

Gaugler, J.E. and Mitchell, L.L. (2022) 'Reimagining family involvement in residential long-term care', *Journal of the American Medical Directors Association*, 23(2), pp. 235–240. Available at: https://doi.org/10.1016/j.jamda.2021.12.022.

92   P. McEvoy et al.

Hall, M. and Sikes, P. (2017) '"It would be easier if she'd died": Young people with parents with dementia articulating inadmissible stories', *Qualitative Health Research*, 27(8), pp. 1203–1214. Available at: https://doi.org/10.1177/1049732317697079.

Hinshelwood, R.D. (1999) 'Countertransference', *The International Journal of Psychoanalysis*, 80(4), pp. 797–818.

Holmes, J. (2018) *A Practical Psychoanalytic Guide to Reflexive Research: The Reverie Research Method*. London: Routledge.

Kessler, D. (2019) *Finding Meaning: The Sixth Stage of Grief*. New York: Scribner.

Kiper, D. (2023) *Travellers to Unimaginable Lands: Dementia, Carers and the Hidden Workings of the Mind*. London: Profile Books Ltd.

Kitwood, T. (1997) *Dementia Reconsidered: The Person Comes First*. Milton Keynes: Open University Press.

Klein, M. (1946) 'Notes on some schizoid mechanisms', *The International Journal of Psychoanalysis*, 27, pp. 99–110.

Lawton, M.P. and Nahemow, L. (1973) 'Ecology and the aging process', in C. Eisdorfer and M.P. Lawton (eds) *The Psychology of Adult Development and Aging*. Washington, DC: American Psychological Association, pp. 619–674.

Lewis, F. et al. (2014) *The Trajectory of Dementia in the UK: Making a Difference*. London: Office of Health Economics Consulting Reports. Available at: www.alzheimersresearchuk. org/wp-content/uploads/2015/01/OHE-report-Full.pdf (accessed 2 February 2024).

Malan, D.H. (1976) *The Frontier of Brief Psychotherapy*. New York: Plenum Press.

McEvoy, P. et al. (2013) 'Empathic curiosity: Resolving goal conflicts that generate emotional distress', *Journal of Psychiatric and Mental Health Nursing*, 20(3), pp. 27–278. Available at: https://doi.org/10.1111/j.1365-2850.2012.01926.x.

Meuser, T.M. and Marwit, S.J. (2001) 'A comprehensive, stage-sensitive model of grief in dementia caregiving', *The Gerontologist*, 41(5), pp. 658–670. Available at: https://doi. org/10.1093/geront/41.5.658.

Mielke, M.M., Vemuri, P. and Rocca, W.A. (2014) 'Clinical epidemiology of Alzheimer's disease: Assessing sex and gender differences', *Clinical Epidemiology*, 6, pp. 37–48. Available at: https://doi.org/10.2147/CLEP.S37929.

Mittelman, M.S., Roth, D.L., Coon, D.W. and Haley, W.E. (2004) 'Sustained benefit of supportive intervention for depressive symptoms in caregivers of patients with Alzheimer's disease', *American Journal of Psychiatry*, 161(5), pp. 850–856. Available at: https://doi. org/10.1176/appi.ajp.161.5.850.

Moore, K.J., Crawley, S., Fisher, E., Cooper, C., Vickerstaff, V. and Sampson, E.L. (2023) 'Exploring how family carers of a person with dementia manage pre-death grief: A mixed methods study', *International Journal of Geriatric Psychiatry*, 38(3), e5867. Available at: https://doi.org/10.1002/gps.5867.

Morris, L. et al. (2020) 'Communication empowerment framework: An integrative framework to support effective communication and interaction between carers and people living with dementia', *Dementia*, 19(6), pp. 1739–1757. Available at: https://doi. org/10.1177/1471301218805329.

Morris, L., Innes, A., Smith, E., Williamson, T. and McEvoy, P. (2021) 'A feasibility study of the impact of a communication-skills course, 'Empowered Conversations', for care partners of people living with dementia', *Dementia*, 20(8), pp. 2838–2850. Available at: https://doi.org/10.1177/14713012211018929.

Nathanson, A. and Rogers, M. (2020) 'When ambiguous loss becomes ambiguous grief: Clinical work with bereaved dementia caregivers', *Health and Social Work*, 45(4), pp. 268–275. Available at: https://doi.org/10.1093/hsw/hlaa026.

Nolan, R., Kirkland, C. and Davis, R. (2021) 'LGBT* after loss: A mixed-method analysis on the effect of partner bereavement on interpersonal relationships and subsequent partnerships', *OMEGA – Journal of Death and Dying*, 82(4), pp. 646–667. Available at: https://doi.org/10.1177/0030222819831524.

ONS (2023) *Monthly Mortality Analysis, England and Wales: March 2023*. London: Office for National Statistics. Available at: www.ons.gov.uk/peoplepopulationandcommunity/

The grief of care partners 93

birthsdeathsandmarriages/deaths/bulletins/monthlymortalityanalysisenglandandwales/
march2023 (accessed 2 February 2024).

Panksepp, J. and Watt, D. (2011) 'What is basic about basic emotions? Lasting lessons from affective neuroscience', *Emotion Review*, 3(4), pp. 387–396. Available at: https://doi.org/10.1177/1754073911410741.

Parkes, C.M. and Prigerson, H.G. (2013) *Bereavement: Studies of Grief in Adult Life*. London: Routledge.

Ramsay-Jones, E. (2019) *Holding Time: Human Need and Relationships in Dementia Care*. Stanmore: Free Association Books.

Ramsay-Jones, E. (2020) *Silly Things*. London: Free Association Books.

Sachdev, P.S. et al. (2014) 'Classifying neurocognitive disorders: The DSM-5 approach', *Nature Reviews Neurology*, 10, pp. 634–642. Available at: https://doi.org/10.1038/nrneurol.2014.181.

Samuel, L.J. et al. (2020) 'Socioeconomic disparities in six-year incident dementia in a nationally representative cohort of US older adults: An examination of financial resources', *BMC Geriatrics*, 20(1), pp. 1–9. Available at: https://doi.org/10.1186/s12877-020-01553-4.

Sellars, M. et al. (2019) 'Perspectives of people with dementia and carers on advance care planning and end-of-life care: A systematic review and thematic synthesis of qualitative studies', *Palliative Medicine*, 33, pp. 274–290. Available at: https://doi.org/10.1177/0269216318809571.

Shay, J. (2014) 'Moral injury', *Psychoanalytic Psychology*, 31, pp. 182–191. Available at: https://psycnet.apa.org/doi/10.1037/a0036090.

Shear, M.K. (2010) 'Complicated grief treatment: The theory, practice and outcomes', *Bereavement Care*, 29(3), pp. 10–14. Available at: https://doi.org/10.1080/02682621.2010.522373.

Taylor, J.S. (2008) 'On recognition, caring, and dementia', *Medical Anthropology Quarterly*, 22(4), pp. 313–335. Available at: https://doi.org/10.1111/j.1548-1387.2008.00036.x.

Tom, S.E. et al. (2015) 'Characterization of dementia and Alzheimer's disease in an older population: Updated incidence and life expectancy with and without dementia', *American Journal of Public Health*, 105(2), pp. 408–413. Available at: https://ajph.aphapublications.org/doi/abs/10.2105/AJPH.2014.301935.

Winnicott, D.W., Winnicott, C.E., Shepard, R.E. and Davis, M.E. (1989) *Psycho-analytic Explorations*. London: Routledge.

Wray, A. and Bergstrom, A. (2023) 'Determiners of social inclusion and exclusion in the dementia context: The perspective of family carers', *Pragmatics and Society*, 23051. Available at: https://doi.org/10.1075/ps.23051.wra.

8 When an adult with significant caregiving responsibilities for children is at end-of-life with cancer

A carer's pre-bereavement and post-bereavement experiences

Jeffrey R. Hanna, Cherith J. Semple, Lisa Strutt

Introduction

This chapter will be presented in two parts:

1. The experience of carers when an adult who has a significant caregiving responsibility for children (<18 years) is at end-of-life with cancer (pre-bereavement).
2. The experience of carers in the first eighteen months after an adult who had a significant caregiving responsibility for children (<18 years) has died with cancer (post-bereavement).

For context, in this chapter the 'carer' is defined as another adult with a significant caregiving responsibility for the children, such as a co-parent. End-of-life is defined as when someone is coming toward the end of their life and are likely to die within the next twelve months (NHS, 2022). The evidence is informed by empirical research studies conducted with adults and children (pre-and-post bereavement), health and social care professionals and funeral directors. There will be insertions from a bereaved parent, Lisa, providing her personal experience of navigating life as a mum to three teenagers (Rosie, James and Holly) and wife (to John) throughout the end-of-life and post-bereavement period.

Part 1 Supporting the family at end-of-life

There are few experiences more difficult for families than preparing children for the death of an adult who has a significant caregiving responsibility for them before adulthood (Hanna, McCaughan and Semple, 2019; Semple et al., 2021). Sadly, this is not an uncommon experience, with one-in-twenty children in the United Kingdom estimated to experience the death of a significant caregiver before adulthood (Childhood Bereavement Network, 2022).

DOI: 10.4324/9781003435365-8

A carer's pre-bereavement and post-bereavement experiences   95

Families are often uncertain how best to prepare and support children for the end-of-life experience of an adult who has a significant caregiving responsibility for them (Pinto and Pinto, 2021). A systematic review of the literature highlighted some key challenges for families telling the children that an adult with a significant caregiving responsibility for them is going to die with cancer (Hanna, McCaughan and Semple, 2019). These included:

- familial beliefs that not telling the children protects them (the children) from pain and upset
- uncertainties about how best to tell the children in a way they would developmentally understand
- opposing familial beliefs about how best the children should be supported; for example, the carer may feel it is in the child's best interest to be informed of the situation, whereas the adult who is dying may feel that not telling the children is protecting them from upset
- uncertainties about the language that is age-appropriate when telling the children that the adult is not going to survive their cancer
- adults' lack of clear understanding of the prognosis themselves
- concerns about difficult questions the children may ask, such as 'when are you going to die?' or 'how are you going to die?'.

Despite children's desire to be informed and involved in the end-of-life experience, many children are not prepared for the expectant death of an adult with cancer who has a significant caregiving responsibility for them (Marshall et al., 2022). Often, children have reported an awareness that 'something is wrong', having observed changes in the home such as more whispered conversations behind closed doors, as well as changes to the unwell adult's physical appearance (Paul, 2019). Children less prepared for the death of an adult who has a significant caregiving responsibility for them are at an increased risk of adverse outcomes in bereavement and later life (Inhestern, Johannsen, and Bergelt, 2021). This includes issues in maintaining and sustaining trusting relationships, a decline in educational attainment, as well as increased risk of substance misuse, criminality, and involvement with mental health services (Birgisdóttir et al., 2023; Høeg et al., 2021). The benefits of open and honest communication in the family at end-of-life are clear, in that they can maintain and sustain the adult-child relationship and mediate for adverse outcomes in bereavement and later life (Eklund et al., 2020).

Families need and want advice and guidance from the healthcare team on how best to prepare and support the children for the end-of-life experience of an adult who has a significant caregiving responsibility for them (Franklin et al., 2019). Health and social care professionals are in an ideal position to provide this important aspect of family-centred cancer care at end-of-life (Dalton et al., 2022; Hanna et al., 2021). The next section will provide further insight to the experience of families at end-of-life, with a key focus on carers and how best they can be supported across the end-of-life continuum.

96 *J.R. Hanna et al.*

Sharing the poor prognosis with the children

Receiving a poor cancer prognosis will be devastating for families and telling the children this news will be at the forefront of the adult's mind. Often, time is required to digest the news before considering telling the children that an adult with a significant caregiving responsibility for them is going to die (Semple et al., 2021). In many families, there can be tension regarding *if* the children should be told about the poor cancer prognosis (Hanna, McCaughan and Semple, 2019). Alongside this, some families may not feel emotionally ready to tell the children that an adult with a significant caregiving responsibility for them is going to die with cancer (Aldridge et al., 2017). For other families, there are often concerns about *how* and *when* is the best time to tell the children, and *what* it is the children should be told about the adult's poor prognosis (Millar, Bell and Casey, 2023; Semple et al., 2022).

> When we received the news of John's terminal diagnosis, Rosie was in the middle of her exams. For the first time in our experience of cancer, John and I decided not to tell the children the news straightaway. When John was first diagnosed with cancer we made a promise to the children – we would always share the information with them unfiltered and first. They could ask any question they wanted to, and we would be as honest and open as possible. We had stayed true to this. The waiting for Rosie's exams to be over was incredibly tough for me and John.

Families want and need advice and guidance about how to tell the children the difficult news that an adult with a significant caregiving responsibility for them is going to die with cancer (Wray et al., 2022a). It is important for health and social care professionals to start the conversations with adults soon after receiving the news of a poor prognosis (Hanna et al., 2021). Often, there is a lack of carer involvement in clinical consultations and appointments, with many feeling on the 'sidelines', ignored by health and social care professionals, and the provision of care centred on the physical needs of the adult who is ill (Semple et al., 2021). Family-centred cancer care is especially important for carers as they are aware that they will have the ongoing caregiving responsibilities for the children after the ill adult has died (Millar, Bell and Casey, 2023). In clinical practice, it is pertinent for the provision of family-centred cancer care to include the needs of carers who have a significant caregiving responsibility for children, such as a mum, dad or grandparent (Hanna et al., 2022).

> Conversations with the healthcare team were centred on John and his care. It probably looked to the health professionals like I was coping very well, because they only see you for a very short time, and the focus was mostly on John. However, there were times when I was struggling to deal with the children - their behaviours and emotions, John's needs and my own. I did initiate some conversations with the clinical nurse specialist about the children when I was particularly worried about them. I did my own research and found a charity who could help teenagers impacted by cancer and I asked the nurse specialist to help me with a referral.

The Talking, Telling, Sharing Framework: End-of-life can provide a useful guide for health and social care professionals as they start conversations with adults about their children (Semple et al., 2022, p. 778). The first part of the framework uses a set of questions as prompts to help open the conversation with adults and assess their attitudes, beliefs and readiness about sharing the poor cancer prognosis with the children. It includes guidance on how to manage familial resistance to telling the children that the adult is going to die with cancer. This includes:

1. acknowledging with adults how difficult these conversations can be;
2. sharing with adults that the children can pick up that 'something is wrong'; and
3. providing the rationale to adults that children cope and adjust better when they are informed and involved.

The second part of the framework helps professionals give guidance to adults on when, where, what, why and how to communicate with the children about the significant caregiver's poor cancer prognosis.

Navigating the end-of-life experience

The end-of-life experience is a changing landscape for families with ongoing and different needs throughout. For families, it is important to strive for everyday ordinariness. This includes maintaining the family routine such as the children going to school and attending their usual extracurricular activities (Fu et al., 2023; Turner, 2020). Often, carers are continuing with work despite the ill adult's declining health. As symptoms progress for the ill adult, often the family adapt and adjust with 'what is happening' as best as possible (Park et al., 2017; Semple et al., 2021).

> Looking back over our family group messages, what I notice is just trying to keep everything moving. My texts are a mix of fact-filled updates from the cancer centre, logistics and calls for the kids to do their chores. You still have the demands of day-to-day living with teenagers and cancer on top. James was swimming competitively then, so I was still getting up at 5.07am each morning to take him to the pool. For him routine was important, so it was very much 'business as usual'. Rosie was exploring university choices, so she focused on working towards that.

Alongside striving for everyday ordinariness, it is important the adults and children have quality time together as a family to facilitate memories for the future (Hanna, McCaughan and Semple, 2019). For families, this is not extravagant activities such as going to Disneyland, but rather 'simple' pleasures that are unique to each family, to include going for a picnic or to the park (Semple et al., 2021). Many carers and children find it helpful taking more photographs, video clips and audio recordings during this period, aiding connectedness to the adult during the post-bereavement period (McCaughan, Semple and Hanna, 2021).

98   *J.R. Hanna et al.*

There were many times during the last year of John's life when we didn't talk about cancer or his impending death. 'Live well to die well' became my driving force. Each of us doing our own thing, as well as sharing family time together. I'm incredibly grateful for these times. Times like going for a walk, a family mealtime, visiting places that meant something to John. Rosie took many selfies and videos with her dad during these times. James watched Star Wars and Marvel movies with him. Holly loved to share all her gaming exploits with John.

It is important for adults to inform and update the child's school of the situation throughout the end-of-life experience. Often, adults find regular updates from the school useful about how the child is coping and reassured that the school will contact them with any concerns about the children (Orr and Henderson, 2020).

Some families may require additional support from healthcare teams as the ill adult becomes physically weak and frailer. For example, facilitating a day out to the child's school sport's day, or having a 'party in the room' to celebrate an occasion if the ill adult is in the acute setting or a specialist palliative care unit (Hanna et al., 2021). This can allow for an everyday family activity to happen, bringing joy to the ill adult, carer and children (Semple et al., 2021). Alongside this, it provides further opportunities for the family to make memories for the future.

There may be occasions throughout the end-of-life experience where adults or children may require additional support and guidance and should be offered a referral to a specialist family support service or psychology services.

Coping as a carer during the unfolding end-of-life experience

The emotions often overwhelm carers as they navigate periods of anticipatory grief, and the harsh reality that the person they may share the closest bond with is going to die, and they will have sole responsibility for the children (Holm et al., 2023). Whilst families strive for everyday ordinariness at end-of-life, this can place added stress on the carer, especially when the ill adult's health deteriorates or if they are admitted to the acute setting (Aamotsmo and Bugge, 2014). At these junctures, the carer is having to navigate key activities alone such as the caregiving for the children and the practical caring needs of the adult who is dying (Semple et al., 2021). Spiritual or religious faith, social networks, and creating time for self-care can be helpful for carers to create balance (Aamotsmo and Bugge, 2014; McCaughan, Semple and Hanna, 2021).

Looking back, the duality of the feelings was something that became ever-present. One minute, simply being glad he was still alive, the next minute experiencing a physical pain in my chest at the thought that he was going to die soon, even though I had no real understanding of what 'soon' meant. I oscillated between just keeping everything moving as 'normal' as possible: mealtimes, activities, chatting, reminiscing, planning, working, updating friends and family, and facing the cold hard reality that he was deteriorating.

A carer's pre-bereavement and post-bereavement experiences   99

Sometimes, it was barely noticeable: a little weight loss, less willingness to take part in family activities and at other times, it seemed to accelerate before my eyes: spasms, irritability, the challenge with finding food John wanted to eat, and trying to get the right combination of meds to alleviate pain.

I coped by having a few close friends to talk to, having a counsellor, writing down my thoughts and feelings, praying, walking, crying when I needed to. There were times where I felt like I was on autopilot, simply and pragmatically doing what had to be done. At other times, I felt the overwhelming sense of foreboding and it was hard to get the motivation to keep going. I found myself setting the morning alarm half an hour before I had to get up for the children and work, just so that I could 'be' in the same space as John [often he was still asleep].

Preparing for the future

It is important for adults to prepare for the future as a supportive means for the family during the end-of-life period, and especially for the carer, moving forward after the death (Bhadelia et al., 2022). This includes outlining funeral wishes, sorting out finances, passwords on accounts, mortgages, or even guardianship for the children. It is important for families to make these preparations when the ill adult is 'well' enough to be able to make decisions (McCaughan, Semple and Hanna, 2021). It is recommended that preparations for the future are made shortly after receiving the poor prognosis, as the ill adult's health may suddenly deteriorate (Breen et al., 2018). Also, earlier preparations can help facilitate quality family time when death becomes imminent, in the final weeks of life (Semple et al., 2021).

For families who do make detailed preparations before the death, carers often feel comforted in that they can fulfil the wishes of the deceased adult (Semple et al., 2021). Also, many carers feel better prepared to navigate life as an adult with sole responsibility for the child's caregiving. For families who do not prepare for the future at end-of-life, carers often experience immense stress and pressures after the ill adult dies, both practically and financially (Hanna and Semple, 2022).

At the time, I frequently talked to John about things I felt he needed to talk to the children about. If I framed it in such a way that it would help me after he died, he seemed to be more motivated to have the conversations. John talked to me about how he knew it would be very hard for me after he died; anticipating the grief of the children and that I would be on my own. I was very appreciative of this because it validated my fears.

Sometimes the pain of having the conversations was suffocating, however I remember a professional saying "he is here now", so that gave me the permission to have the difficult conversations, hug him, cry and appreciate that he was still alive in that moment.

We talked about the life we had had together: the highs and lows, what was important to him in terms of his funeral, expectations for me and the children immediately and long-term. We left no stone unturned regarding the

100   *J.R. Hanna et al.*

conversations. There is no doubt in my mind that these conversations have helped me in my grief and my ability to continue living life after John died.

Often, healthcare teams encourage the ill adult to engage in memory activities such as writing letters for the future or making memory boxes, to aid the child's connectedness following the adult's death (Franklin et al., 2019; Wray et al., 2022a). However, in post-bereavement, many carers have reported struggling with the appropriate timing of providing these to the children. In some situations, adults have died before they had time to complete letters or write one for each of their children (Hanna and Semple, 2022). Rather, talking about the adult that died, and looking at the photos and videos that were taken in the family before the cancer, and throughout the end-of-life period facilitates connectedness for the carer and children (Hansen et al., 2016; Semple et al., 2021). While some families find it helpful to engage in memory activities, it is important for professionals to realise that a 'one size fits all' approach is not helpful, as this can place additional pressure on the ill adult pre-bereavement (Semple et al., 2021), and the carer post-bereavement (Hanna and Semple, 2022).

Navigating the final weeks of life

Often there is a point in the ill adult's illness when their body will no longer respond to treatment and there is an evident decline in their health. This timepoint will vary for ill adults. There will be some ill adults that may be clinging to hope at this point for treatment to extend life. However, the carer is often more realistic that death is becoming imminent, having observed an overall decline in the ill adult's health (Semple et al., 2021). Despite this, carers are often shocked at how hasty death approached, not fully appreciating they are 'running out of time' (Semple et al., 2021).

> I had taken Rosie to visit a University in London and returned home to find a John whose sparkle had diminished – he was very ill, and I knew it. John was in the dying phase. No one told us that. I asked because it was getting harder and harder to meet his needs. At that time, we still had the nurse come once a week. I was doing all the caring. John didn't get out of bed much. It was hard for the kids to know how to be with him.
>
> One evening John felt very unwell and was hospitalised (one month before he died). I thought I wouldn't see him again. I believe an opportunity was missed at this stage to explain to us how far along he really was in terms of end-of-life.

Whilst many carers are aware that the ill adult's health is deteriorating, many are unaware that death is imminent, as they often have not, or rarely have, experienced the death of a close relative (Mannix, 2018). There is a need for professionals to take a lead on an important conversation with adults, that death is imminent and, where appropriate, provide realistic timescales (Mannix, 2021).

> From the news of the terminal diagnosis until the final weeks of life, I always had an eye on the end. I was not in denial; however, I did not know what

would happen to him physiologically and what was fast or slow in terms of deterioration. John was very independent, particularly regarding personal hygiene, and he had always been physically strong. A tell-tale sign for me that he was very ill was when he took a bath to relieve pain in his back (about four weeks before he died): he did not have the strength to get himself out of the bath and I could not get him out myself, so I had to call upon my son to help. This was a significant milestone.

As death becomes more imminent in the final weeks of life, it is important to encourage adults to tell the children that the ill adult's treatment is no longer working, and death is approaching (Hanna et al., 2021; Marshall et al., 2021; Muñoz Sastre, Sorum and Mullet, 2016). For many families, it is often the carer who is now navigating key conversations with the children alone, as often the ill adult is too poorly to be part of them (Semple et al., 2021). Also, some ill adults find it too difficult to be part of these emotional conversations (McCaughan, Semple and Hanna, 2021). It is important that the adults explain what dying means to children and that they understand it as a permanent state (Marshall et al., 2022).

In the final weeks of life, the carer is often focused on spending time with the ill adult and attending to their care needs. Often, the children appear to be on the sidelines at this point, and the significant adult caregivers are less well connected to the children (Semple et al., 2021). To navigate this period, it is important for health and social care professionals to encourage carers to maximise available support networks to help with the practical elements of parenting and to alleviate pressures (McCaughan, Semple and Hanna, 2021). This can include taking and collecting the children from school or helping with household chores.

John was adamant that I cared for him and that he wanted to be at home as long as possible. I felt the pressure of his wishes and the limitations of my ability to care properly for him. One of the biggest challenges for me at this time was his medicines regime – it was constantly changing in response to his increased pain and discomfort. As the carer, I felt like I had to advocate for John as he often wasn't able to / didn't want to articulate the true extent of his pain.

He was increasingly frustrated with how he was feeling and the ineffectiveness of the pain management. I was juggling work, John's care and the children's needs. By this stage, I was still working but up every three to four hours during the night to administer medication.

Navigating the final days of life

Many families are often uncertain when the death is expected to happen (Semple et al., 2021). It is helpful when health and social care professionals provide this honest information and prepare carers by explaining the physiological aspects of dying (Mannix, 2018). This includes changes to breathing such as becoming more irregular, with slow and deep, rapid or noisy breaths, as well as changes to the person's pallor. Also, explaining that once the adult has died their body will become cold to touch.

I didn't really understand the physiological aspects of death and dying. I had to ask. I was grateful when the palliative consultant explained what would happen physiologically, and how there was no clear timescale. She gave me signs to look out for and helped me to simply be present in the time I had.

Carers are often uncertain what involvement children should have in the final days of life. Where possible, carers should be encouraged to give children the choice to be present when the adult is dying (Fearnley and Boland, 2017). Children have highlighted their desire to have the opportunity to 'say goodbye' to the adult (Hanna, McCaughan and Semple, 2019; Marshall et al., 2022). Many children may 'dip in and out' of the room, spending time with the adult in the final days of life. This can provide the children with the opportunity to hold the adult's hand and tell them how much they love them. While the adult who is dying may not be able to answer the children, it is important for the carer to reassure the children that the adult can often still hear them (Sheehan et al., 2014). Like with adults, it is important to explain to children the physiological aspects of dying (Hanna and Semple, 2022). Telling younger children that the adult will no longer need to eat or drink when they die can help to explain the permanency of death (Sheehan et al., 2014).

Part 2 Supporting the carer in bereavement

Following the death, the family transition to the immediate bereavement period. This is the period between the death happening and the funeral taking place, where there are key religious and spiritual events for the carer and children. The timing of this period varies for families and is often impacted by cultural and religious practices, as well as the uniqueness of each family's situation. One of the greatest challenges facing the carer is what role the children will have at this time (Hanna, McCaughan, and Semple, 2022). Often, carers have reflected it would have been helpful to have considered the children's role in the immediate bereavement period before the ill adult died (Hanna and Semple, 2022).

It is important that children are given the opportunity to be part of the immediate bereavement period, to aid their understanding of death and to feel part of the family (Faro, 2018). This can include the listening to and sharing of stories of the adult that died, choosing the outfit of the adult that died, the flowers or music for the funeral, and taking part in the funeral service (Hanna, McCaughan and Semple, 2022). In some cultures, the funeral director has been highlighted as instrumental in guiding and supporting carers through the immediate bereavement period and encouraging involvement of the children in cultural, religious or spiritual activities (Hanna, McCaughan and Semple, 2022; Mahon, 2009). The immediate bereavement period can be a 'busy' time for many carers, with an increase in visitors coming to the home and finalising the funeral plans.

Following the immediate bereavement period, there can be a period of major transition for carers, which can impact on the family's routine, available social networks and relationships (Wray et al., 2022b). After the death of an adult who had a significant caregiving responsibility for children, often the carer is now having to navigate their own grief, that of the children's and the caregiving responsibilities

A carer's pre-bereavement and post-bereavement experiences   103

of the children alone (McClatchey, 2018; Shorey and Pereira, 2023). This section will provide insight of the carers' experience after the funeral, and how best they can be supported in bereavement. While the experiences for individual carers will vary, the evidence below is predominately reflective of the first eighteen months after the funeral.

Adjusting to life as a sole carer

For carers and children, it is helpful for the children's routine to continue shortly after the funeral to provide security and stability (Duncan, 2020; Harrop et al., 2022). This includes the children going back to school and being part of their usual extracurricular activities (Hanna and Semple, 2022). For some carers, this can be challenging, especially if they are now taking on the caregiving responsibilities that may have traditionally been led by the deceased adult with cancer (Holmgren, 2021). Some carers strive to be 'perfect' and aim to maintain the aspects of everyday life that were typical for the family before the ill adult died (Shorey and Pereira, 2023). This can place immense stress and pressure on the carer in the early days after the death, with many feeling exhausted and overwhelmed, as they navigate their own and the children's grief, as well as the caregiving responsibilities for the children alone (Hanna and Semple, 2022). It is important for carers to be encouraged to practice self-care so that they can meet the needs of their children (Eklund et al., 2022). Although not always available, it can be helpful for carers to be encouraged to maximise social networks to help with the practical aspects of caregiving from close family members and friends, such as taking the children to school or helping with household chores (Wray et al., 2022b). Carers often find this to be a great source of relief and facilitates more quality time together as a family in the evenings and weekends (Hanna and Semple, 2022).

> Immediately after John died, I was hit by a wall of fatigue. I slept an inordinate amount of time. I would see the children out to school, then sleep, sometimes not getting up until just before they arrived home. John died in October, so the next big milestone was Christmas and I resolved to make it as special as possible. It was Holly's 16th birthday on Christmas Day. That kept me going. A friend met me on Fridays to walk and talk. I found this helped me get through the emptiness of the weekends.

Loneliness is often an intense feeling experienced by carers in the post-bereavement period. This includes navigating aspects of caregiving alone and making key decisions as a sole carer, such as choosing a secondary school for the children (Hanna and Semple, 2022; Shorey and Pereira, 2023). Some carers with older children (>13 years) often report more time at home alone, as teenage children often prefer to spend time with friends (Tillquist, Bäckrud and Rosengren, 2016). Also, carers often have a strong sense of missing aspects of life, particularly in activities that were previously cherished as a family or couple (Hanna and Semple, 2022; Wray et al., 2022b).

I frequently found myself eating alone, which exacerbated the suffocating sense of loneliness and loss. The children retreated to their bedrooms and often didn't want to participate in family mealtimes. I found this hurtful at times, especially as it had always been an integral part of our family life. Sometimes I enforced a family mealtime, but a mix of respecting the children's wishes and simply being too tired for a fight meant that I accepted it.

Navigating the grief experience as a carer with children

Grief is a subjective experience that will vary between and within families (Kumar, 2023). Like adults, the grief experience will vary for children with periods of sadness, upset and anger (Parsons, Botha and Spies, 2021). Some carers find it helpful to access counselling. It is important for carers to understand that children may not grieve in the expected way, with emotions such as crying. Children can experience periods of upset or anger in situations outside of the home, for example at school or during their extracurricular activities (McManus and Paul, 2019). It is helpful for carers to be informed by the child's school or other key adults in the child's life if there are concerns regarding their wellbeing (Hanna and Semple, 2022).

Having three children, I have seen how individual the grief experience is: from not talking about it, to anger, frustration and needing additional support. I had a good relationship with the school but for Holly, attending school was a daily challenge in the months immediately following John's death.

Carers often feel they have to 'keep it together' for the children by not sharing with them how they are coping in their grief (McClatchey, 2018). Nonetheless, carers reflect it is helpful when informed that telling the children how they are feeling can facilitate opportunities for the children to share with the carer how they are coping (Angelhoff et al., 2021; Hanna and Semple, 2022). In doing so, this can enable adult-child support during their grief experience (Shorey and Pereira, 2023). Alongside this, carers and children find it helpful to talk about the adult that died to keep their memory alive (Hansen et al., 2016). This is often facilitated through looking at the photos, video and audio clips that were taken as a family before the adult died (Hanna and Semple, 2022).

We have a family WhatsApp group and I often post pics of the good family times. Things, like, 'this time last year, we were here . . .'. I think this helped give the children permission to share memories. Rosie had captured many videos of her dad and she frequently shared them too. James and Holly less so, and they found it more difficult to talk about him.

Meeting other families who have experienced similar situations can be helpful for carers to hear the 'stories' of how others navigated their grief (McClatchey, 2018; Shorey and Pereira, 2023). Also, gleaning tips as to how other carers navigated elements of family life as a sole caregiver for the children (Hanna and

A carer's pre-bereavement and post-bereavement experiences   105

Semple, 2022). It can be helpful for the children to meet other children who have experienced similar situations to know they are not alone in this journey (Bugge et al., 2014). Meeting others is often facilitated through family support services (Wray et al., 2022b). Often, families stop accessing these services around eighteen months as they do not feel they are 'in the same place' as new families who start to attend (Hanna and Semple, 2022).

> We benefited greatly from support from a local cancer charity. We attended events up to two years after John died where we met other families in bereavement. I believe that because we had talked so much about life after death when John was still alive, the children found themselves 'further on' than other children in their grief journeys. Rosie has gone on to volunteer for a charity as a childhood bereavement ambassador.

'Giving back' is often helpful for carers after the adult has died with cancer, such as fundraising for cancer charities (McClatchey, 2018). Also, carers feel it is honouring the legacy of the adult that died to tell their 'story' to others, promoting a positive impact for future families who find themselves in this unfortunate situation (Hanna and Semple, 2022).

> I am on a board of a cancer charity, and I regularly give talks about cancer, death and dying. This is important to me as it helps tell our story, honours John's legacy and makes me feel that some good can come out of this devastating experience. I have found it extremely encouraging to know that I have helped others by sharing our story. I believe if we can do something to better the end-of-life experiences I want to be at the heart of that.

In summary: 'Don't forget the carer'

Children are a key concern for families when an adult with a significant caregiving responsibility for children is at end-of-life with cancer. Families are often unsure how best to support the children at end-of-life and post-bereavement. Children less involved in the end-of-life and post-bereavement experience are at increased risk of adverse outcomes in later life. Carers are often navigating key conversations with the children alone, such as telling them the adult is going to die, preparing for the dying experience, and the events that will take place in the immediate bereavement period. Also, after the adult's death, carers are often overwhelmed with having to navigate the children's and their own grief, as well as the caregiving responsibilities for the children. It is pertinent that the provision of family-centred care is provided to carers at end-of-life and post-bereavement to facilitate better outcomes for the whole family.

> Just because someone looks like they are coping, doesn't mean they are all the time. One thing I learned is how quickly the caring landscape changes. It's okay for health and social care professionals to probe a little deeper,

106   *J.R. Hanna et al.*

check for understanding, ask what has changed since the last time and ultimately to provide a safe space to explore how the carer is with their caring responsibilities. Even if the professional feels they are not the person who can help the carer, they should at least be able to signpost to other support.

References

Aamotsmo, T. and Bugge, K.E. (2014) 'Balance artistry: The healthy parent's role in the family when the other parent is in the palliative phase of cancer – challenges and coping in parenting young children', *Palliative and Supportive Care*, 12(4), pp. 317–329. Available at: https://doi.org/10.1017/S1478951513000953.

Aldridge, J. et al. (2017) 'I can't tell my child they are dying: Helping parents have conversations with their child', *Archives of Disease in Childhood: Education and Practice*, 102(4), pp. 182–187. Available at: https://doi.org/10.1136/archdischild-2016-311974.

Angelhoff, C. et al. (2021) 'Communication, self-esteem and prolonged grief in parent-adolescent dyads, 1–4 years following the death of a parent to cancer', *European Journal of Oncology Nursing*, 50, p. 101883. Available at: https://doi.org/10.1016/j.ejon.2020.101883.

Bhadelia, A. et al. (2022) 'Identifying core domains to assess the "quality of death": A scoping review', *Journal of Pain and Symptom Management*, 63(4), pp. e365–e386. Available at: https://doi.org/10.1016/j.jpainsymman.2021.11.015.

Birgisdóttir, D. et al. (2023) 'Family cohesion predicts long-term health and well-being after losing a parent to cancer as a teenager: A nationwide population-based study', *Plos One*, 18(4), p. e0283327. Available at: https://doi.org/10.1371/journal.pone.0283327.

Breen, L.J. et al. (2018) 'Family caregivers' preparations for death: A qualitative analysis', *Journal of Pain and Symptom Management*, 55(6), pp. 1473–1479. Available at: https://doi.org/10.1016/j.jpainsymman.2018.02.018.

Bugge, K.E. et al. (2014) 'Young children's grief: Parents' understanding and coping', *Death Studies*, 38(1), pp. 36–43. Available at: https://doi.org/10.1080/07481187.2012.718037.

Childhood Bereavement Network (2022) *Key statistics*. London: Childhood Bereavement Network. Available at: https://childhoodbereavementnetwork.org.uk/about-1/what-we-do/research-evidence/key-statistics (accessed 10 May 2023).

Dalton, L.J. et al. (2022) 'Exploring healthcare professionals' beliefs, experiences and opinions of family-centred conversations when a parent has a serious illness: A qualitative study', *Plos One*, 17(11), e0278124. Available at: https://doi.org/10.1371/journal.pone.0278124.

Duncan, D.A. (2020) 'Death and dying: A systematic review into approaches used to support bereaved children', *Review of Education*, 8(2), pp. 452–479. Available at: https://doi.org/10.1002/rev3.3193.

Eklund, R. et al. (2020) 'The family talk intervention for families when a parent is cared for in palliative care: Potential effects from minor children's perspectives', *BMC Palliative Care*, 19(1), pp. 1–10. Available at: https://doi.org/10.1186/s12904-020-00551-y.

Eklund, R. et al. (2022) 'Talking about death when a parent with dependent children dies of cancer: A pilot study of the Family Talk Intervention in palliative care', *Death Studies*, 46(10), pp. 2384–2394. Available at: https://doi.org/10.1080/07481187.2021.1947415.

Faro, L.M. (2018) 'When children participate in the death ritual of a parent: Funerary photographs as mnemonic objects', *Religions*, 9(7), 215. Available at: https://doi.org/10.3390/rel9070215.

Fearnley, R. and Boland, J.W. (2017) 'Communication and support from health-care professionals to families, with dependent children, following the diagnosis of parental life-limiting illness: A systematic review', *Palliative Medicine*, 31(3), pp. 212–222. Available at: https://doi.org/10.1177/0269216316655736.

A carer's pre-bereavement and post-bereavement experiences   107

Franklin, P. et al. (2019) 'Health and social care professionals' experiences of supporting parents and their dependent children during, and following, the death of a parent: A qualitative review and thematic synthesis', *Palliative Medicine*, 33(1), pp. 49–65. Available at: https://doi.org/10.1177/0269216318803494.

Fu, C. et al. (2023) 'A qualitative systematic review about children's everyday lives when a parent is seriously ill with the prospect of imminent death: Perspectives of children and parents', *OMEGA - Journal of Death and Dying*. Available at: https://doi.org/10.1177/00302228221149767.

Hanna, J.R. et al. (2022) 'Conversations about children when an important adult is at end of life: An audit', *American Journal of Hospice and Palliative Medicine*, 39(7), pp. 806–811. Available at: https://doi.org/10.1177/10499091211046241.

Hanna, J.R. et al. (2021) 'Providing care to parents dying from cancer with dependent children: Health and social care professionals' experience', *Psycho-Oncology*, 30(3), pp. 331–339. Available at: https://doi.org/10.1002/pon.5581.

Hanna, J.R., McCaughan, E. and Semple, C.J. (2019) 'Challenges and support needs of parents and children when a parent is at end of life: A systematic review', *Palliative Medicine*, 33(8), pp. 1017–1044. Available at: https://doi.org/10.1177/0269216319857622.

Hanna, J.R., McCaughan, E. and Semple, C.J. (2022) 'Immediate bereavement experiences when a parent of dependent children has died of cancer: Funeral directors' perspectives', *Death Studies*, 46(4), pp. 969–978. Available at: https://doi.org/10.1080/07481187.2020.1793433.

Hanna, J.R. and Semple, C.J. (2022) 'I didn't know what was in front of me: Bereaved parents' experience of adapting to life when a co-parent of dependent children has died with cancer', *Psycho-Oncology*, 31(10), pp. 1651–1659. Available at: https://doi.org/10.1002/pon.6010.

Hansen, D.M. et al. (2016) 'Parental relationships beyond the grave: Adolescents' descriptions of continued bonds', *Palliative and Supportive Care*, 14(4), pp. 358–363. Available at: https://doi.org/10.1017/S1478951515001078.

Harrop, E. et al. (2022) 'Parental perspectives on the grief and support needs of children and young people bereaved during the COVID-19 pandemic: Qualitative findings from a national survey', *BMC Palliative Care*, 21(1), p. 177. Available at: https://doi.org/10.1186/s12904-022-01066-4.

Høeg, B.L. et al. (2021) 'Psychotropic medication among children who experience parental death to cancer', *European Child and Adolescent Psychiatry*, 32, pp. 155–165. Available at: https://doi.org/10.1007/s00787-021-01846-y.

Holm, M. et al. (2023) 'How parents of dependent children reason about their partner's impending death due to cancer', *Death Studies*, 47(1), pp. 105–110. Available at: https://doi.org/10.1080/07481187.2021.1992807.

Holmgren, H., (2021) 'Life came to a full stop: The experiences of widowed fathers', *OMEGA - Journal of Death and Dying*, 84(1), pp. 126–145. Available at: https://doi.org/10.1177/0030222819880713.

Inhestern, L., Johannsen, L.M. and Bergelt, C. (2021) 'Families affected by parental cancer: Quality of life, impact on children and psychosocial care needs', *Frontiers in Psychiatry*, 12, 765327. Available at: https://doi.org/10.3389/fpsyt.2021.765327.

Kumar, R.M. (2023) 'The many faces of grief: A systematic literature review of grief during the COVID-19 pandemic', *Illness, Crisis and Loss*, 31(1), pp. 100–119. Available at: https://doi.org/10.1177/10541373211038084.

Mahon, M.M. (2009) 'Funeral directors and bereaved children: Beliefs and experiences', *Death Studies*, 33(9), pp. 828–847. Available at: https://doi.org/10.1080/07481180903142464.

Mannix, K. (2018) *With the End in Mind: Dying, Death, and Wisdom in an Age of Denial*. London: Harper Collins Publishers.

Mannix, K. (2021) *Listen: How to Find the Words for Tender Conversations*. London: Harper Collins Publishers.

Marshall, S. et al. (2021) 'The perspectives of children and young people affected by parental life-limiting illness: An integrative review and thematic synthesis', *Palliative Medicine*, 35(2), pp. 246–260. Available at: https://doi.org/10.1177/0269216320967590.

Marshall, S. et al. (2022) 'It's not just all about the fancy words and the adults: Recommendations for practice from a qualitative interview study with children and young people with a parent with a life-limiting illness', *Palliative Medicine*, 36(8), pp. 1263–1272. Available at: https://doi.org/10.1177/02692163221105564.

McCaughan, E., Semple, C.J. and Hanna, J.R. (2021) 'Don't forget the children: A qualitative study when a parent is at end of life from cancer', *Supportive Care in Cancer*, 29(12), pp. 7695–7702. Available at: https://doi.org/10.1007/s00520-021-06341-3.

McClatchey, I.S. (2018) 'Fathers raising motherless children: Widowed men give voice to their lived experiences', *OMEGA – Journal of Death and Dying*, 76(4), pp. 307–327. Available at: https://doi.org/10.1177/0030222817693141.

McManus, E. and Paul, S. (2019) 'Addressing the bereavement needs of children in school: An evaluation of bereavement training for school communities', *Improving Schools*, 22(1), pp. 72–85. Available at: https://doi.org/10.1177/1365480219825540.

Millar, R., Bell, M. and Casey, L. (2023) 'The struggle between protecting children from and preparing them for the death of their parent: A qualitative study', *American Journal of Hospice and Palliative Medicine*, 40(5), pp. 539–543. Available at: https://doi.org/10.1177/10499091221111560.

Muñoz Sastre, M.T., Sorum, P.C. and Mullet, E. (2016), 'Telling children their mother is seriously ill or dying: Mapping French people's views', *Child: Care, Health and Development*, 42(1), pp. 60–67. Available at: https://doi.org/10.1111/cch.12270.

NHS (2022). *What End of Life Care Involves*. London: National Health Service. Available at: www.nhs.uk/conditions/end-of-life-care/what-it-involves-and-when-it-starts/ (accessed 13 September 2023).

Orr, D. and Henderson, M. (2020) 'Talking to children about death, dying and bereavement: Is it time for a change in the school curriculum?', *British Journal of Child Health*, 1(3), pp. 117–119. Available at: https://doi.org/10.12968/chhe.2020.1.3.117.

Park, E.M. et al. (2017) 'Parenting while living with advanced cancer: A qualitative study', *Palliative Medicine*, 31(3), pp. 231–238. Available at: https://doi.org/10.1177/0269216316661686.

Parsons, A., Botha, J. and Spies, R. (2021) 'Voices of middle childhood children who lost a mother', *Mortality*, 26(1), pp. 1–16. Available at: https://doi.org/10.1080/13576275.2019.1696291.

Paul, S. (2019) 'Is death taboo for children? Developing death ambivalence as a theoretical framework to understand children's relationship with death, dying and bereavement', *Children and Society*, 33(6), pp. 556–571. Available at: https://doi.org/10.1111/chso.12352.

Pinto, C. and Pinto, S. (2021) 'When a parent is dying: How we can do more to support families and children with a dying parent', *Evidence-Based Nursing*, 24(1), 4. Available at: https://doi.org/10.1136/ebnurs-2019-103192.

Semple, C.J. et al. (2021) 'Living in parallel worlds - bereaved parents' experience of family life when a parent with dependent children is at end of life from cancer: A qualitative study', *Palliative Medicine*, 35(5), pp. 933–942. Available at: https://doi.org/10.1177/02692163211001719.

Semple, C.J. et al. (2022) 'Parent's with incurable cancer: Nuts and bolts of how professionals can support parents to communicate with their dependent children', *Patient Education and Counseling*, 105(3), pp. 775–780. Available at: https://doi.org/10.1016/j.pec.2021.06.032.

Sheehan, D.K. et al. (2014) 'Telling adolescents a parent is dying', *Journal of Palliative Medicine*, 17(5), pp. 512–520. Available at: https://doi.org/10.1089/jpm.2013.0344.

Shorey, S. and Pereira, T.L.B. (2023) 'Parenting experiences of single fathers: A meta-synthesis', *Family Process*, 62(3), pp. 1093–1113. Available at: https://doi.org/10.1111/famp.12830.

Tillquist, M., Bäckrud, F. and Rosengren, K. (2016) 'Dare to ask children as relatives! A qualitative study about female teenagers' experiences of losing a parent to cancer', *Home Health Care Management and Practice*, 28(2), pp. 94–100. Available at: https://doi.org/10.1177/1084822315610104.

Turner, N. (2020) 'My life's properly beginning: Young people with a terminally ill parent talk about the future', *Sociology of Health and Illness*, 42(5), pp. 1171–1183. Available at: https://doi.org/10.1111/1467-9566.13086.

Wray, A. et al. (2022a) 'Parental terminal cancer and dependent children: A systematic review', *BMJ Supportive and Palliative Care*, 0, pp. 1–13. Available at: https://doi.org/10.1136/bmjspcare-2021-003094.

Wray, A. et al. (2022b) 'Parental death: A systematic review of support experiences and needs of children and parent survivors', *BMJ Supportive and Palliative Care,* 36384696. Available at: https://doi.org/10.1136/spcare-2022-003793.

9 When caring ends

Exploring the hidden aspects of loss in trajectories out of caring in Australia

Emma Kirby, Giselle Newton, Louisa Smith, Iva Strnadová, Brendan Churchill, Lukas Hoffstätter, Sarah Judd-Lam, and Christy E. Newman

Introduction

Irrespective of the informal caring context, caring, at some point, inevitably comes to an end. The circumstances of how caring ends may vary: others may take over caring duties, the condition of the person being cared for may improve, or caring may end in bereavement. While carers' experiences are diverse and varied, caring trajectories inevitably entail a range of processes and experiences, through which a considerable proportion of carers become *former carers* (Cavaye and Watts, 2016; Corey and McCurry, 2018; Kirby et al., 2022; Larkin, 2009; Larkin and Milne, 2021). Through a range of processes and various aftereffects of caring, former carers have been shown to experience manifold impacts in terms of their wellbeing, including poor health outcomes, social isolation, and financial precarity. Yet, end-of-caring experiences have received relatively little research attention (Larkin and Milne, 2021). In response, a burgeoning scholarship has foregrounded former carers' experiences, and futures planning, as simultaneously crucial to the project of conceptualising (and better supporting) trajectories out of caring (Cavaye and Watts, 2016; Larkin, 2009; Walker and Hutchinson, 2019; Watts and Cavaye, 2018). Extending this work, in this chapter we explore experiences of loss within trajectories out of caring in Australia. As we will discuss, pathways out of caring can be difficult to navigate, complicated by multiple and layered forms of loss, and inflected by social and cultural expectations related to post-caring life.

Informal carers in Australia

There are over 2.6 million informal carers in Australia (Australian Bureau of Statistics, 2020). This means that approximately 10 percent of the population is engaged in the provision of unpaid care and support to a family member or friend who has a disability, mental illness, drug and/or alcohol dependency, chronic condition, terminal illness, or who is frail (Carers NSW 2020; see also the Carer Recognition Act 2010 [Cth], s 5). In Australia, the most common care is that provided to a spouse or

DOI: 10.4324/9781003435365-9

partner, child, or parent. Carers are more likely to be female, middle-aged, and on average provide 35 hours of caring per week (ABS, 2020). Given the demands of informal caring – physically, emotionally, and temporally – it is unsurprising that carers have significant need for social, health and economic support (Australian Institute of Health and Welfare, 2019; Cresswell, 2017). In the Australian context, federal and state-funded government supports exist to provide training, peer support, counselling services and respite, and income benefits, according to the individual care circumstances (Cresswell, 2017; AIHW, 2019). Since 2020, many of these services have been integrated via the Carer Gateway service model (Department of Social Services, 2021), an Australian Government program that provides free services and support for carers (although several services are still provided through other means, for example aged care and disability services). Carer Gateway also provides resources and personal stories to help carers; these include topics such as preparing and planning for the end of life and planning for the future. The availability of services and support across Australia, however, varies – as does engagement with such services.

When considering support for transitions out of caring in Australia, the *Carer Recognition Act* (2010) outlines how carers should be supported, and includes provisions for wellbeing, employment, and education. The Act refers specifically to timely, appropriate, and accessible support for carers; however, it does not include specific reference to former carers. Indeed, former carers (or carers transitioning out of their caring roles) tend to receive only incidental attention across policy and service support. Instead, former carers tend to fall into other categories: for example, carers as bereaved people may access entitlements to (limited) payment or allowance following a person's death (Social Security Act, 1991 [Cth], s 21). Former carers may also fall into the category of 'job seeker' and, as such, receive government payments allocated to those actively looking for paid work. What emerges is a landscape within which carers have been shown to experience a 'post-caring void' (Larkin and Milne, 2021).

What makes a 'care ending'?

How care endings are understood and recognised, has important implications for practice as well as scholarly debates. Several questions emerge: How do we know when caring is coming to an end? How and in what ways can (and should) we delineate *current* from *former* or *ex*-carers? When do care endings begin and end? Here, we use 'care endings' as a term to describe the full range of contexts and experiences in trajectories from the 'active' phase of caring to the 'post-caring' period (Kirby et al., 2022). Existing research has outlined various *care endings*, including: the relinquishment of full-time care via admission of the care recipient into supported accommodation; the recovery or improvement (however partial) of the care recipient's condition; or bereavement (Cavaye and Watts, 2016; Davies and Nolan, 2004; Larkin and Milne, 2021; Watts and Cavaye, 2018). In day-to-day caring life, endings are likely to be experienced as complicated and fraught with

112   E. Kirby et al.

challenges. The point at which a *current* carer becomes a *former* carer, for example, is rarely clear cut. This lack of temporal clarity is often revealed in prolonged caring commitments, where the duties of caring, and the carer identity, can continue long after the caring role may be assumed to have ended (Cavaye, 2006; Larkin and Milne, 2021; Molyneaux et al., 2011). Carers may also move in and out of caring roles, according to fluctuating requirements over the life course (Larkin, 2009); this means frequent and/or transient experiences of 'endings'. Research has shown the prevalence of caring for multiple recipients concurrently, where the end of caring for one recipient may not in itself signal an end to caring overall (Carers NSW, 2020). Indeed, experiences of caring (whether current or former) also rely on carers' identification with their role: sometimes people in caring roles do not identify as a *carer*; rather, as a parent, a child, a partner, a supportive friend, and so on (Molyneaux et al., 2011). As such, their experience may be rendered less visible in terms of recognition from the state, and/or from their social networks.

How are trajectories out of caring experienced? Grief, loss, visibility and recognition

A key aspect of trajectories out of caring is the affective, private process of making sense of changes as caring ends. Research internationally has revealed experiences of grief and loss in bereavement, as well as loss of identity, sense of self, and purpose, as carers navigate life beyond caring (Cronin et al., 2015; Davies and Nolan, 2004; Larkin, 2009; Nathanson and Rogers, 2020). Bereavement is perhaps the most visible context in which caring ends. Following the death of a loved one, carers must navigate experiences of grief at a time when their day-to-day caring duties, roles, and identities are shifting. Studies have illustrated the impacts of bereavement on the emotional wellbeing of carers, including the relationship between care-related stressors before bereavement and post-bereavement psychological support needs (Aneshensel, Botticello and Yamamoto-Mitani, 2004). The importance of the relationship between caregivers' pre-death grief and distress and post-death adjustment has long been foregrounded, particularly in terms of the need for health services and support for bereaved caregivers (Breen, 2012). Several scholars have pointed to the need for greater attention to bereaved carers' needs as they (re)construct their lives beyond caring (Breen, 2012; Kirby et al., 2018; Larkin, 2009).

Another prominent context is the (re)location of caring – where informal carers may relinquish primary responsibility for the care recipient, as they move to hospital, aged care, or other supported accommodation. Research across settings shows that carers experience various challenges within these transitions, particularly in coming to terms with having less control or decision-making agency, as well as feelings of guilt related to relinquishing care. Dahlborg Lyckhage and Lindahl (2013), for example, in the context of transitions to palliative care, highlighted how carers live in liminality, as simultaneously visible and invisible vis-à-vis formal, professional care (see also Davies and Nolan, 2004). In the context of dementia, several studies have revealed the difficulties faced by former carers in coping with separation, particularly in feelings of connection, obligation, and uncertainty (Corey and McCurry, 2018; Egdell, 2013).

When caring ends 113

Although the circumstances may vary, there is evidence across settings of the 'aftereffects' of caring for former carers. These *effects* may be, in part, due to taking on a caring role in the first place, and/or may continue, or intensify, after caring ends. Research has highlighted poorer health, including fatigue and burnout, as well as delayed diagnoses of illness in contexts where carers may compromise their own wellbeing to prioritise that of the care recipient (Cronin et al., 2015; Larkin, 2009; Watts and Cavaye, 2018). In addition, former carers have been shown to experience lingering effects of depression, loneliness and social isolation (see also Kirby, van Toorn and Lwin, 2022). In the Australian National Carer Survey, for example, Hawthorn Friendship Scale scores indicated that 48 percent of carers remained socially isolated after their caring ends (Carers NSW, 2022). In addition, almost 45 percent of former carers reported experiencing at least one form of financial stress (Carers NSW, 2022). Other Australian research has detailed the negative impacts of having a caring role on long-term income, lifetime savings and the superannuation balance at retirement age (Furnival and Cullen, 2022). As such, experiences of caring coming to an end inevitably entail aspects of *loss*. Loss can come in many forms: for example, research shows widespread unmet needs among former carers, including gaps in support and service provision (Orzeck and Silverman, 2008; Watts and Cavaye, 2018). Moreover, and as we explore in the case study below, we see many less visible examples of loss. These experiences shape the transition from caring and post-caring identities, including in carers' attempts to 'move on' following caring coming to an end. Such examples are wide ranging, for instance from (re)entering the labour market, managing finances to support retirement, to fostering social relationships and identity in terms of imagined futures.

Case study: Carers' attitudes to and experiences of trajectories out of caring

In what follows, we explore the experiences and perspectives of a group of carers based in New South Wales, Australia, who participated in a series of focus group discussions in 2022. The focus groups consisted of young carers (18–30), carers who self-identified as 'current' carers who were thinking or had considered how their caring role may come to an end, and those who identified as 'former' carers (but who may indeed still be engaged in the work of caring or identify with a carer identity). Each group comprised between three and five discussants, lasted between 60 and 150 minutes, and were guided by a schedule of discussion topics. The carers spanned a range of caring contexts and relationships, including caring for parents, young children and adult-aged children, siblings, partners, and friends. All but one of the carers were female. Some carers chose to discuss the specificities of the recipients' care needs, while others did not. During the focus groups we were cognisant not to ask for details related to a care recipient's condition to foreground privacy and sensitivity to carer and recipient circumstances. Broadly speaking, caring circumstances related to ageing, frailty and dementia, mental health difficulties, children with additional needs, physical disability, and acquired brain injury. Most participants had at least three years'

114   *E. Kirby et al.*

experience in their caring role; some had been carers for decades. Of those who identified as former carers, caring ended for two participants in bereavement, for two participants in the transition of caring to residential aged care, one had moved away (to attend university), and one participant described their status as 'currently not required' in the context of episodic caring duties. For the analysis that follows, we thematically coded the focus group transcripts, informed by the interpretive traditions within sociology, and focused on reaching a comprehensive and nuanced understanding of the various positions and perspectives of participants, situated within systems of beliefs and experiences more broadly (Charmaz, 2006). The lead author independently systematically read through each focus group transcript, taking notes, followed by discussion of these notes and ideas with two other authors. Through this iterative process, we identified patterns within the data, whilst trying to retain the complexity and nuances of participants' accounts (Ezzy, 2002).

Making sense of loss as caring ends: Loss, expectation, obligation, and guilt

The first 'hidden' aspects of loss we focus on relate to how cultural and relational expectations for caring shape how caring ends. Across the focus groups, participants described their commitment to *doing caring well*. As such, they were often worried, or ambivalent, about the sustainability of caring, and the need to adjust as their caring ended. As one participant said:

> I'm sad and I'm scared about the thought of not being my child's carer anymore. I understand it needs to happen, and it will happen and that's great, that's healthy, that's normal. But it's going to be a huge loss . . . most of my identity is as a carer. I'm proud of it. I think I've done a great job. And I've built my jobs around caring. So, I'll also have to adjust.

Several current and former carers described how difficult they found it to talk about or plan for their caring to end, for fear it might be perceived as 'giving up' on the care recipient, or as indicative of them 'not caring enough'. Care endings were sometimes reflected on as a *failure* on the part of the carer, perhaps reflecting assumptions that the carer had not made enough effort to sustain their caring or did not have the skills required. These accounts were often grounded in normative pressures to continue caring. For example, one participant said:

> [There is] this cultural expectation to always be there, always care. Taking a break or leaving means you don't love them.

This and other accounts revealed constructs of caring as a 'labour of love' and show how social norms, related to familial traditions or expectations, can affect carers (Egdell, 2013; Keating, 2019). Discussions often turned to how such expectations were not universal – affecting how the work of caring is unevenly distributed within families (in turn including variation in carer's ability to transition out of their caring role):

I've looked at moving out . . . but then I feel guilty. But then at the same time. I get jealous of my brother because he was able to move out. I'm just like, I'm just stuck. And like, I feel bad for feeling that.

Here we see feelings of guilt that were threaded through each group's discussions. This personal, private management of complicated feelings – of guilt, obligation, envy, and loss of 'good' caring identity – were talked about by several participants, revealing how the *virtues* of caring are culturally elevated. As one said:

No matter how long you are a carer for, there is always a feeling of guilt at one point or another.

In this way, a good carer might be one who neither anticipates nor desires their caring to end. Another participant talked about the tendency for carers to self-sacrifice, as a means of proving their dedication to caring (see also Kirby, van Toorn and Lwin, 2022), something that was then difficult to resolve as caring ends:

I look back and I go, what the hell was I doing? I'm really proud of myself. But I know at that time I thought I needed to do more and more to prove to myself that I can keep up with everyone else as well as being a carer.

Managing these experiences was isolating for carers, who felt that the emotions often embedded in 'moving on' from caring were taboo, and likely to be judged by others. In this way, relationships felt lost, where relational distance was an inevitable consequence of feeling unable to *open up* about the emotions of care endings. A good example of this was the relief, and/or freedom, felt by some participants as they transitioned into life beyond caring:

I've noticed there's that sudden . . . . Like I wouldn't say freedom, but I do have a little bit of extra time. And so, it's just reestablishing what that time is and what I can do with that time. And that's been . . . it's been interesting.

Here, the reestablishing of 'extra time' is imbued with feelings of freedom and of guilt. For some, this meant that life beyond caring seemed impossible:

You get to the stage where you want to transition out of care, like it to end, but you just can't.

116   *E. Kirby et al.*

For other participants, however, endings were possible, likely, but difficult to predict:

> When my child gets quite well, then my caring role finishes. But then when they get unwell the role comes back. It's not something that's sort of final, it's something that's sort of quite ambiguous.

This uncertainty made it difficult for carers to plan their futures. In such cases, we heard several accounts of carers grieving for opportunities lost, for example:

> I'm starting to feel that life is passing me by, that I'm not able to do the things I would like to do or go to the places I would like to visit. I listen to other people talk of their experiences and I am starting to feel envious.

We next turn our attention to accounts of lost opportunities in more depth, in exploring how experiences of grieving for lost pasts and lost futures reveal themselves as caring ends.

Grieving lost pasts and lost futures

Across the focus groups, participants described how becoming a carer meant that their life trajectories, opportunities, and sense of self, had shifted in various ways that could not be seen, and were often not recognised by others. Most commonly we heard about missed professional and financial opportunities, which were couched by all participants as losses:

> I gave up my career eight years or so ago. There's no way I can get back into it. I'm too far behind now, I'd have to do a lot of study to catch up.

Another participant commented:

> There's not really much support for carers returning to work when you're mid-career. So how do you re-skill or up skill to get back to that level that you are at where you left?

Importantly, the striation of workforce participation according to existing structural inequities (particularly gender and age – the excerpts above and below are from middle-aged women), is seen here in accounts of lost opportunities and lost futures (Ehrlich, Möhring and Drobnič, 2020; Furnival and Curren, 2022; Spijker et al., 2021). The time spent outside the labour market also had consequences for the ways in which participants perceived their financial stability in life beyond caring:

> I'm in the midst of my career. I'm at the peak of my earning capacity right now. And so that's something that really does weigh on me. It hasn't altered my decision to be a carer, or to be working part time. But I still see how I am

When caring ends   117

impacted now. And also, you know, in my future I know my superannuation [pension] is nothing like my peers.

Another participant shared how the skills she had developed as a carer lacked visibility and recognition in her life after caring. In addition to these losses, for this participant, the absence of a tenancy history was another practical and emotional challenge:

> I was applying for homes to move into. It was so difficult because they would ask 'what's your tenancy history?' I don't have one, but as a carer I've had to manage a household, finances, responsibilities, retirement, and superannuation – this should make me an ideal tenant.

Lost opportunities were reflected in considerable uncertainties, particularly related to the future. Caring roles prompted profound changes in participants' future imaginaries, threatening carers' sense of ontological security. One participant, a woman in her thirties, caring for a parent, shared how the ways by which she conceptualised life in the future had fundamentally shifted, to become more responsive to uncertainty and change:

> I've become much more apprehensive about my future. Because seven years ago I didn't think I'd be here like this is, it's a reasonably short amount of time.. . . It's not negative in any way, but it's just shown me that in such a short amount of time my life is nowhere near where I thought it would be. I don't know where it's going to be in another seven years either . . . . I just know that there's so much that I'm kind of unprepared for, which I'm not as worried about right now, I think that's one attribute caring has really given me – that things shift. So, I'm much more accepting of change, especially if it's not something that I've chosen. And so, I think that whilst I'm apprehensive about my future because there is a lot of uncertainty, I'm not as worried as I maybe would have been a few years ago.

Similarly, another participant – currently transitioning out of her caring role – reflected on the uncertainty of her imagined future, balancing longer-term hope with more immediate fears:

> So, I can see a really rosy future. But if I think about this month, or this year or next year that freaks me out.

What was clear across the focus groups was that a lack of preparedness contributed to such uncertainties, especially in experiences of loss:

> Nobody prepares you for, in the health system, for the carer ending process and you're kind of left in the lurch like this about finding grief processes, grief counselling services or support groups on your own terms.

118   E. Kirby et al.

This lack of preparedness resonates with the findings of existing research on anticipation and bereavement, particularly in showing how grief and bereavement affects carers' psychological and social wellbeing (e.g., Aneshensel, Botticello and Yamamoto-Mitani, 2004; Breen, 2012; MacArthur, Kirby and Mowll, 2023).

Moving on? Care endings, (lack of) support, and (loss of) belonging

Here we turn to participants' accounts of what Corey and McCurry (2018) term 'learning to live again' after caring ends. Participants' experiences in many ways reflected the vulnerabilities former carers experience in terms of their marginalised position within policy and service provision. In Australia, as in many high-income countries, support and entitlements tend to focus on current or 'active' carers, rather than those deemed to be 'post-caring' (Larkin and Milne, 2021; Orzeck and Silverman, 2008). In this way, support (from government, but also from social networks and communities more broadly) was viewed by several participants as *lost* within trajectories out of caring, despite ongoing needs. For some, there was a sense of abandonment and injustice, as one participant described:

> So, it's [caring is] coming in, it's doing it, and then suddenly you dropped off the edge down here to flounder and there's no preparation for that.

We heard many examples of what has been called the 'post-caring void' (Larkin and Milne, 2021). We find this concept of the void particularly useful here, as it at once can encapsulate an absence of support, and an absence of recognition. These absences imply an imperative for carers to 'move on' as their caring ends, to engage in the work of building a new post-caring identity, role and purpose. What we heard from participants were the challenges inherent to learning to live again without practical and material support. Not only did endings require mental and emotional scope to plan, they also required specific economic conditions:

> Basically, you don't have the financial resources to be able to transition out of [caring], into something else.

The issue of belonging, of being categorised as a 'carer' (and therefore entitled to government support) relative to a 'former carer' (lacking such entitlements) was discussed at length within the focus groups. Participants rarely knew which way to turn for support. For example, one participant pointed to how it felt counterintuitive to seek advice about pathways out of caring from organisations designed to sustain and support their role as carers:

> It seems strange, I suppose I could talk to [carer support service]. . . to call to say (that) I'm moving out of caring, how do I do that?

When caring ends 119

Others shared their frustrations at the lack of structural support for trajectories out of caring, framed within logics of social justice and fairness:

> Even though I've given up my relationships and my career, etc, there's still that voice and I think that's a societal voice and a family voice saying 'but you should, you better, you must . . .'. Who's going to help me when I'm no longer looking after my son, in a really practical, tangible sense, with my ailing health, no family nearby, income, housing. So, do I become homeless?

The loss of a sense of belonging experienced by several former carers was exacerbated by this lack of structural support. Significant bureaucratic barriers were talked about by participants, as impeded access to recognition. Several participants, like the one below, highlighted the entanglement of societal recognition, funding provision, and (a lack of) belonging for former carers:

> So, these are the [online] portals they are like the sieves or funnels that we want people to go through. And if you don't fit in that funnel, or if you don't fit within that category, then you don't get funding, you don't get the recognition as well.

This excerpt was indicative of feelings of lost identity; what Scott (2020) describes as "a state of *not-having* something that had once defined herself" (p. 173). Further, this account revealed uncertainty in trajectories out of caring, which we saw through accounts that questioned whether, when, and how, carers would 'find themselves again'. Such difficulties, of making sense of manifold losses without clear recognition or support, were further complicated for those in circumstances where government entitlements had been withdrawn, but the everyday toll of caring remained. For example, the participant below was struggling to manage everyday life amidst transition:

> Because Mum is moving into permanent care, I don't get that [government support] package. Even though I'm still providing her emotional support, support with all the administrative stuff.. . . It's a lot, it's really time consuming, helping mum to navigate those systems. It's transitioning the role and there's still support I need.

Conclusion

In this chapter we have sought to contribute to the growing literature oriented towards making visible the broader inequities and vulnerabilities of (former) carers. In doing so we aimed to foreground how loss is socially and relationally regulated (Jakoby, 2015). Through the accounts of a group of Australian carers, we have shown some of the ways that losses are unrecognised and hidden. Given the wealth of research

120   E. Kirby et al.

that evidences how informal caring lacks visibility, it is unsurprising, then, that navigating trajectories out of caring – including the various and diverse losses that carers must grieve – also lacks visibility and recognition. We have also shown how loss is experienced differentially, according to socio-cultural expectations and moralities that circulate around caring. As opportunities to mobilise alternative caring arrangements vary, so too do opportunities for some carers to extricate themselves from caring roles, or (re)enter careers or social relationships (Dahlberg, Demack and Bambra, 2007; Egdell, 2013). Our case study also reveals how some losses are felt and experienced as more legitimate, and perhaps more grievable – than others (see also Fowlkes, 1990; Butler, 2009). This is particularly the case in accounts of loss of direction, loss of self, and loss of purpose, experienced by former carers (Larkin and Milne, 2021; cf. Charmaz, 1983). Moreover, we see the challenges experienced by many carers in coping with a lack of recognition on the part of social networks and institutions, prompting a loss of faith or trust in communities. The injustice experienced by carers in our research was clear, particularly in their awareness of a lack of identification or acknowledgement of former carers, despite the profound reliance on carers to help sustain health and social care systems (Williams, 2012). In addition, our participants felt the imperative to 'move on', to transition from *good* carers to *good* citizens, to actively seek a life after caring (see also Addo et al., 2021). Without support for, and recognition of, hidden forms of loss, many more carers are likely to find themselves in the post-caring void, where a lack of belonging may prolong or exacerbate poorer health and wellbeing. More attention in research and policy is needed to rethink and improve service provision tailored to the needs of former carers, across a range of caring relationships and contexts.

References

ABS (2020) *Disability, Ageing and Carers, Australia: Summary of Findings, 2018*. Canberra, Australia: Australian Bureau of Statistics. Available at: www.abs.gov.au/statistics/health/disability/disability-ageing-and-carers-australia-summary-findings/latest-release (accessed 5 February 2024).

Addo, I.Y. et al. (2021) 'Young carers in Australia: Understanding experiences of caring and support-seeking behaviour', *Australian Social Work*, 77(1), pp. 60–73. Available at: https://doi.org/10.1080/0312407X.2021.1971271.

Aneshensel, C.S., Botticello, A.L. and Yamamoto-Mitani, N. (2004) 'When caregiving ends: The course of depressive symptoms after bereavement', *Journal of Health and Social Behavior*, 45(4), pp. 422–440. Available at: https://doi.org/10.1177/002214650404500405.

AIHW (2019) *Informal Carers*. Canberra, Australia: Australian Institute of Health and Welfare. Available at: www.aihw.gov.au/reports/australias-welfare/informal-carers (accessed 5 February 2024).

Breen, L.J. (2012) 'The effect of caring on post-bereavement outcome: Research gaps and practice priorities', *Progress in Palliative Care*, 20(1), pp. 27–30. Available at: https://doi.org/10.1179/1743291X12Y.0000000003.

Butler, J. (2009) *Frames of War: When is Life Grievable?* London: Verso.

Carers NSW (2020) *2020 National Carer Survey: Summary Report*. Sydney, Australia: Carers New South Wales. Available at: www.carersnsw.org.au/research/survey (accessed 5 February 2024).

Carers NSW (2022) *National Carer Survey 2022 Report*. Sydney, Australia: Carers New South Wales. Available at: www.carersnsw.org.au/about-us/our-research/carer-survey (accessed 5 February 2024).

When caring ends 121

Cavaye, J. (2006) *Hidden Carers*, volume 3. Edinburgh: Dunedin Academic Press.

Cavaye, J. and Watts, J.H. (2016) 'Former carers: Issues from the literature', *Families, Relationships and Societies*, 7(1), pp. 141–157. Available at: https://doi.org/10.1332/20467 4316X14676464160831.

Charmaz, K. (1983) 'Loss of self: A fundamental form of suffering in the chronically ill', *Sociology of Health and Illness* 5(2), pp. 168–195. Available at: https://doi.org/ 10.1111/1467-9566.ep10491512.

Charmaz, K. (2006) *Constructing Grounded Theory: A Practical Guide through Qualitative Analysis*. London: Sage Publications.

Corey, K.L. and McCurry, M.K. (2018) 'When caregiving ends: The experiences of former family caregivers of people with dementia', *The Gerontologist*, 58(2), pp. e87–96. Available at: https://doi.org/10.1093/geront/gnw205.

Cresswell, A. (2017) 'Collateral damage: Australian carers' services caught between aged care and disability care reforms', *International Journal of Care and Caring*, 1(2), pp. 275–279. Available at: https://doi.org/10.1332/239788217X14951899318122.

Cronin, P. et al. (2015) 'Between worlds: The experiences and needs of former family carers', *Health and Social Care in the Community*, 23(1), pp. 88–96. Available at: https://doi.org/10.1111/hsc.12149.

Dahlberg, L., Demack, S. and Bambra, C. (2007) 'Age and gender of informal carers: A population-based study in the UK', *Health and Social Care in the Community*, 15(5), pp. 439–445. Available at: https://doi.org/10.1111/j.1365-2524.2007.00702.x.

Dahlborg Lyckhage, E. and Lindahl, B. (2013) 'Living in liminality – being simultaneously visible and invisible: Caregivers' narratives of palliative care', *Journal of Social Work in End-of-Life and Palliative Care*, 9(4), pp. 272–288. Available at: https://doi.org/10.1080 /15524256.2013.846885.

Davies, S. and Nolan, M. (2004) 'Making the move': Relatives' experiences of the transition to a care home', *Health and Social Care in the Community*, 12(6), pp. 517–526. Available at: https://doi.org/10.1111/j.1365-2524.2004.00535.x.

Department of Social Services (2021) *Integrated Carer Support Service Model*. Canberra, Australia: Department of Social Services. Available at: www.dss.gov.au/disability-and-carers-carers/ integrated-carer-support-service-model (accessed 5 February 2024).

Egdell, V. (2013) 'Who cares? Managing obligation and responsibility across the changing landscapes of informal dementia care', *Ageing and Society*, 33(5), pp. 888–907. Available at: https://doi.org/10.1017/S0144686X12000311.

Ehrlich, U., Möhring, K. and Drobnič, S. (2020) 'What comes after caring? The impact of family care on women's employment', *Journal of Family Issues*, 41(9), pp. 1387–1419. Available at: https://doi.org/10.1177/0192513X19880934.

Ezzy, D. (2002) *Qualitative Analysis: Practice and Innovation*. London: Routledge.

Fowlkes M.R. (1990) 'The social regulation of grief', *Sociological Forum*, 5(4), pp. 635–652. Available at: www.jstor.org/stable/684689.

Furnival, A. and Cullen, D. (2022) *Caring Costs Us: The Economic Impact on Lifetime Income and Retirement Savings of Informal Carers*. Turner, Australia: Carers Australia. Available at: /www.carersaustralia.com.au/wp-content/uploads/2022/04/Caring-Costs-Us_Summary-of-Findings_FINAL_070422.pdf (accessed 4 February 2024).

Jakoby, N.R. (2015) 'The self and significant others: Toward a sociology of loss', *Illness, Crisis and Loss*, 23(2), pp. 129–174. Available at: https://doi.org/10.1177/1054137315575843.

Keating, N., Eales, J., Funk, L., Fast, J. and Min, J. (2019) 'Life course trajectories of family care', *International Journal of Care and Caring*, 3(2), pp. 147–163. Available at: https:// doi.org/10.1332/239788219X15473079319309.

Kirby, E. et al. (2018) 'The meaning and experience of bereavement support: A qualitative interview study of bereaved family caregivers', *Palliative and Supportive Care*, 16(4), pp. 396–405. Available at: https://doi.org/10.1017/s1478951517000475.

Kirby, E. et al. (2022) '(How) will it end? A qualitative analysis of free-text survey data on informal care endings', *International Journal of Care and Caring*, 6(4), pp. 604–620. Available at: https://doi.org/10.1332/239788221X16357694113165.

Kirby, E., van Toorn, G. and Lwin, Z. (2022) 'Routines of isolation? A qualitative study of informal caregiving in the context of glioma in Australia', *Health and Social Care in the Community*, 30, pp. 1924–1932. Available at: https://doi.org/10.1111/hsc.13571.

Larkin, M. (2009) 'Life after caring: The post-caring experiences of former carers', *The British Journal of Social Work*, 39(6), pp. 1026–1042. Available at: www.jstor.org/stable/23724130.

Larkin, M. and Milne, A. (2021) 'Knowledge generation and former carers: Reflections and ways forward', *Families, Relationships and Societies*, 10(2), pp. 287–302. Available at: https://doi.org/10.1332/204674319X15761550214485.

MacArthur, N.D., Kirby, E. and Mowll, J. (2023) 'Bereavement affinities: A qualitative study of lived experiences of grief and loss', *Death Studies*, 47(7), pp. 836–846. Available at: https://doi.org/10.1080/07481187.2022.2135044.

Molyneaux, V., Butchard, S., Simpson, J. and Murray, C. (2011) 'Reconsidering the term "carer": A critique of the universal adoption of the term "carer"', *Ageing and Society*, 31(3), pp. 422–437. Available at: https://doi.org/10.1017/S0144686X10001066.

Nathanson, A. and Rogers, M. (2020) 'When ambiguous loss becomes ambiguous grief: Clinical work with bereaved dementia caregivers', *Health and Social Work*, 45(4), pp. 268–275. Available at: https://doi.org/10.1093/hsw/hlaa026.

Orzeck, P. and Silverman, M. (2008) 'Recognizing post-caregiving as part of the caregiving career: Implications for practice', *Journal of Social Work Practice*, 22(2), pp. 211–220. Available at: https://doi.org/10.1080/02650530802099866.

Scott, S. (2020) 'The unlived life is worth examining: Nothings and nobodies behind the scenes', *Symbolic Interaction*, 43(1), pp. 156–180. Available at: https://doi.org/10.1002/symb.448.

Spijker, J.J.A. et al. (2021) 'What factors enable mid-life carers to re-enter the labour market in New Zealand?', *Australasian Journal on Ageing*, 40, pp. 154–161. Available at: https://doi.org/10.1111/ajag.12852.

Walker, R. and Hutchinson, C. (2019) 'Care-giving dynamics and futures planning among ageing parents of adult offspring with intellectual disability', *Ageing and Society*, 39(7), pp. 1512–1527. Available at: http://doi.org/10.1017/S0144686X18000144.

Watts, J.H. and Cavaye, J. (2018) 'Being a former carer: Impacts on health and well-being', *Illness, Crisis and Loss*, 26(4), pp. 330–345. Available at: https://doi.org/10.1177/1054137316679992.

Williams, C. (2012) 'Chronic illness and informal carers: 'Non-persons' in the health system, neither carers, workers or citizens', *Health Sociology Review*, 21(1), pp. 58–68. Available at: https://doi.org/10.5172/hesr.2012.21.1.58.

10 Former carers

Grief, loss and other stories

Mary Larkin and Alisoun Milne

Introduction

Although the growing number of carers – in the UK and internationally – is now widely acknowledged, it is much less recognised that there is also a growth in the number of those who were carers: a population known as 'former carers'. In the UK, it is estimated that around a third of carers become former carers each year. Despite the fact that this group is now achieving some (limited) academic and public recognition, they are largely invisible in carer-related research and policy (Larkin and Milne, 2021; Milne and Larkin, 2023).

Whilst the vast majority of research on caring focuses on the active phase(s) of care (i.e., care provided in the community by the family carer), there is a developing body of work on former carers. Research remains limited in both quantity and quality, but it has led to greater understanding of the distinctive status of former carers and some of the different dimensions of their experiences (Cavaye and Watts, 2018; Larkin and Milne, 2021).

Beginning with a brief discussion of definitional issues relating to the term former carer, this chapter will then explore what is known about former carers' grief and loss. How work on this important issue can be extended to increase understanding is the focus of our final section. Whilst every effort has been made to include international literature, for reasons of brevity and consistency, examples of policy, services and practice are UK-based. Although the terms 'caregiving' and 'caregiver' tend to be favoured more in US-based research, the terms 'carer', 'caring' and 'former carer' are used throughout the chapter.

Who is a former carer?

The former carers field is characterised by considerable terminological inconsistency. This can be attributed to two main factors. The first is that the concept of 'former carer' is drawn from the wider concept of 'carer', which despite being relatively embedded in policy and public discourse, is still a contested term and status. The fact that 'carer' is not recognised or owned as a descriptive label by as many as half of those who actually do caring is an influential factor (Lloyd, 2006; Molyneaux et al., 2011; Milne and Larkin, 2023). That carers do

DOI: 10.4324/9781003435365-10

not belong under *one* definitional umbrella and are a diverse population also contributes to its differential usage. Further complexity arises in relation to some groups of carers too. Older carers with their own physical health problems for example, may be simultaneously a service user *and* a carer supporting a partner with dementia (Rapaport and Manthorpe, 2008; Larkin, Henwood and Milne, 2022).

The second source of confusion arises from evidence that there is more than one route into acquiring the status of former carer. Cavaye and Watts (2018) highlight two of the most common routes – when the cared-for person is admitted to a care home or when they die. Other routes include when the cared-for person is admitted to a hospital or hospice, s/he goes into remission (e.g., for cancer patients), and s/he recovers from their health problem (e.g., those who have undergone major surgery) (Larkin and Milne, 2017).

Being a former carer is not necessarily a static state either. Carers may transition in and out of being a carer and then a former carer across their life course. For example, a woman may care for her parent and then some years later for her husband. In between those roles she is a former carer. This has been termed 'serial caring' (Seltzer and Li, 2000; Larkin, 2009). The increasing demand for family care across and within generations means that more and more people are likely to be serial carers – and former carers – in the future (Carers UK, 2019).

Loss of caring role and identity

Whatever route carers take into post-caring life and however frequently they transition from being a carer into being a former carer, they face the loss of their caring role upon each transition. Research carried out to date suggests that the loss of this role is complex as it is linked to a wide range of emotional responses which encompass: distress; loss of self-esteem and sense of purpose; negative feelings such as anger, guilt, disorientation and emptiness; disconnection with those they had come to know through being a carer (e.g. other carers); and a sense of failure. The strength of, and interrelationships between, these emotional responses often means that former carers can find it difficult to adapt to not being a carer anymore (i.e., to a non-caring role). Hence, finding a new way to 'be' and a new identity are key challenges for many former carers (Larkin and Milne, 2017; Cavaye and Watts, 2018).

The losses and challenges take different forms for different groups of former carers as well as for different individuals. For the increasing number of serial carers, the end of a caring role does not represent a permanent loss. Although they may feel they have little choice in taking on another caring role, as somebody who is closely related to them needs care, lost caring roles are replaced with other caring roles. For those who are not serial carers and for whom the loss of their caring role is more permanent, there is evidence that carer identity shapes the post-caring identities of carers of those admitted to a care home and bereaved carers. It is to this evidence we now turn.

Former carers 125

Box 10.1   Case study: Jane's story

Iris had become increasingly forgetful since she reached the age of 80; she was also becoming frail. Whilst she was able to live in her own home, her eldest daughter – Jane – over a period of about ten years, had gradually been providing more and more support for her mother as her memory got worse and her mobility decreased. During her last two years at home, Jane was granted power of attorney and arranged for carers to visit once a day to help with Iris' personal care and ensure her safety when Jane was unavailable because of work and other commitments. When it got to the point where Iris could not be left for more than an hour on her own, Jane very reluctantly reached the conclusion that she should use Iris' savings to pay for her to move into a care home. Jane visited Iris every other day, often sitting in the lounge with her and chatting to other residents and staff. When Iris raised any concerns (e.g., about her care, other residents, how staff had treated her), Jane would pursue these with the care home manager. She also attended any social events organised at the care home and ran a weekly art class for the residents. Jane routinely went through Iris' wardrobe and sorted out her clothes for each day. When Iris had a very heavy cold and could not get out of bed, she gave her a bed bath and saw to her toileting needs.

Carers of those admitted to a care home for long-term care, especially if they are a spouse carer, may struggle with the implications of this life-changing decision for their role and status both within and outside the home. Although admission inevitability involves a transfer of (some) responsibility for care from the carer to the care home staff, as the case study about Iris and Jane illustrates, carers often remain involved in care activities albeit in a 'new' formulation of the caring role (Larkin and Milne, 2021). This role often includes: visiting their relative regularly; advocating for them; interacting with other residents, relatives and staff; taking part in social events; and monitoring the quality of care. It may also involve continuing to provide some of their previous care tasks (e.g., helping their relative with bathing, offering emotional support, and managing their money). At a more nuanced level, former carers routinely carry out a range of performative roles such as helping staff to understand the character, life and identity of their relative based on their life course and biographical knowledge; this is especially important if the person has dementia (Kirby et al., 2022; Larkin and Milne, 2021). Continuing to care has been found to improve carers' sense of self and identity, although adopting a new identity is harder for some carers, such as male spousal dementia carers (Milne and Hatzidimitriadou, 2003). This may, in part, be explained by the fact that older husbands tend to struggle more than older wives to re-engage with interests or friends once caring has ended. It is largely a gendered distinction (Larkin, 2009).

126   M. Larkin and A. Milne

Studies on carers who become former carers because the person they cared for dies show that some bereaved carers, particularly those who have been caring intensively and over the longer term, continue to be involved in some level or type of caring role or activity post-caring. This may include: helping friends or neighbours with daily tasks; doing paid care work; undertaking voluntary work (such as committee work) associated with caring; continuing to be involved with a carers group or a carers centre; and/ or maintaining social networks that have been developed during the caring journey. It is no coincidence that many of those who work in third sector carers agencies have been carers themselves (Larkin, 2009; Cronin et al., 2015; Larkin and Milne, 2021).

Grief

Some of the ways carers are challenged by the loss of their carer role and identity with the transition of the cared-for person to a care home were referred to above. There is also evidence (Cronin et al., 2015) that the transition itself is accompanied by feelings of loss and grief; carers often feel that they have failed to 'do enough' to keep their relative at home. It is important to note the influence of the broader context in which decisions to seek admission to a care home are located. Carers can be very sensitive to negative perceptions of institutional care; they often view the placement of a relative as challenging the dominant paradigm of 'home' as the best site of care and a care home as a 'last resort'. These perceptions can increase existing feelings of guilt which may be further compounded in situations where carers are not confident that they have secured the best placement for their relative (Cronin et al., 2015).

When the cared-for person dies, bereavement can be harder for carers than non-carers and have longer term emotional consequences (Cavaye and Watts, 2018). Although some report feeling a sense of satisfaction that 'they did everything they could for their relative', most reactions are negative (e.g., stress, depression characterised by shock, numbness, pain, intense sorrow, anger and distress). A number of influences on bereaved carers' emotional wellbeing have been identified. Interestingly, the wellbeing of carers whose relative is admitted to a care home and subsequently dies appears to improve to a greater degree than carers whose relative dies in the community (Larkin and Milne, 2021). This finding may be explained by the fact that carers whose relative is in a care home may have come to terms with a number of the psychological challenges associated with bereavement (e.g., separation, loneliness, loss) *before* their relative actually dies. Other protective factors include: being present at the death; having had a close relationship with the care recipient; good family functioning; having a higher level of self-esteem; emotional support; and higher levels of education and income. In contrast, higher levels of distress among bereaved carers appear to be linked to specific negative care-related influences such as: reluctance to be a carer; emotional strain; role overload; lack of support during caring; caring for someone who experienced high levels of suffering (e.g., a cancer patient); and dissatisfaction with caring (Larkin, 2009; Cavaye and Watts, 2018).

Work exploring the complexities of carer bereavement has identified the concept of 'anticipatory loss' (Eloniemi-Sulkava et al., 2002; Hughes, Locock and

Former carers 127

Ziebland, 2013). This focuses on the fact that carers often experience many years of 'losing' their relative before death; this most often applies to caring for someone with dementia. Other losses include loss of freedom and hopes for the future. This process can give rise to a multitude of conflicting emotions, both during caring and after death (Larkin and Milne, 2021).

A related concept is that of 'anticipatory grief'. This term has been employed specifically in relation to dementia carers; the gradual loss of cognitive and physical function eventually results in what some commentators call 'social death' of the person living with dementia. Carers mourn the loss of the person they knew before dementia. 'Anticipatory grief' – unlike 'anticipatory loss' – is evidenced as *preparing* or even *protecting* carers from some of the negative effects of bereavement itself (Greenwood and Smith, 2019). That dementia carers are often exposed to this 'two-stage bereavement' process may also explain why they report higher levels of improved wellbeing post death and over the long term compared with other groups of bereaved carers (Cavaye and Watts, 2018).

Finally, any discussion of carer loss and grief should not overlook the fact that some former carers – irrespective of their route into their status as a former carer – feel a sense of great relief when they are no longer caring. This is particularly the case for those carers who have been subjected to physical, emotional, verbal or sexual coercion and/or aggression, whether this behaviour is intentional or unintentional (as in dementia), from the cared-for person. Studies show that carers are disinclined to disclose what is happening to them when they are experiencing harm because they fear their relative being 'removed' to a care home or that they would be condemned for 'not coping' (Spencer et al., 2019; Isham, Bradbury-Jones and Hewison, 2020, 2021). Their anxiety can be compounded by the fact that their experiences contradict the public and policy narrative about family care being wholly positive and virtuous and that all carers are good at providing care. Some, mainly female, carers may have been exposed to domestic abuse for many years; becoming a carer may overlay a pre-existing pattern of abuse (Milne, 2023). Living with such fears can lead to carers adopting defensive coping strategies, such as emotional containment and minimisation of contact with family and friends as well as services and professionals. This, in turn, deepens carers' level of isolation and social detachment, issues which are explored in the next section.

The 'legacies of caring'

Box 10.2   Case study: Robinder's story

Robinder's wife, Preeti, suffered from multiple sclerosis for over twenty years. Although Robinder was unable to take up any offer of promotion, because his caring role did not allow him to devote more time to work, he managed to work in the earlier stages of his wife's illness. The impact of the multiple sclerosis on Preeti's physical and mental wellbeing meant they did less and less outside the home and their social circle dwindled to a few family members only. Despite some local authorty funding, Robinder ended up using most of their savings on specialist equipment that would improve Preeti's quality of life and reduce the exhausting demands of caring on him. When she died, the exhaustion caught up with him and he had a complete breakdown which included debilitating depression from which he never fully recovered. Unable to work, Robinder was reliant on benefits and had little spare income with which to rebuild a social life. His relatives became very worried about his increasing reclusivity and organised a 'rota' so that they took it in turns to take him out on a weekly basis.

The preceding discussions of carer grief illustrate the influence of losses experienced *during* caring on carers' *post caring* lives. There are many other losses associated with caring itself that intersect with the post caring trajectory for carers who are bereaved; these are often referred to as the 'legacies of caring' (Larkin, 2009; Larkin and Milne, 2017). Some of these are illustrated in Robinder and Preeti's story above. When caring ceases, many carers are left with significant financial losses; this is a consequence of the combined impact of additional care-related expenses (e.g., extra laundry and higher heating bills) and carers having to work reduced hours or give up work altogether. Attenuated labour market participation reduces income both at the time and, because of reduced pension contributions, in retirement. Carers' financial challenges are compounded by the loss of their carer-related benefits once 'active' caring ends. Few former carers report an improvement in their finances post-caring. In part, this is because post-caring opportunities to address financial losses can be very limited even for those of working age. Work-related skills and professional and social networks lost during caring can damage prospects of returning to a pre-caring job or embarking on a new career post-caring (Cronin et al., 2015; Cavaye and Watts, 2018).

Some of the losses experienced by carers in relationship to paid work are mirrored in carers' social worlds too. For the vast majority of carers, particularly those who care over the long-term, there is a contraction of their social networks and interests. Most carers have reduced levels of social activity during their caring 'career' and do not have the time or money to pursue interests. This is, perhaps obviously, linked to another legacy of caring – social isolation and loneliness; studies indicate that as many as 80 percent of carers are lonely and that loneliness levels persist well into their post-caring lives (Robinson-Whelan et al., 2001; Carers UK, 2021; Geerlings et al., 2022).

In addition, caring has a well-established link with creating, or deepening, existing physical and psychological health problems. These often persist into, and may even worsen, post-caring. Such health issues include back problems, exhaustion, depression, distress, skin disorders, infections, arthritis, high blood pressure and cardiac problems (Cronin et al., 2015; Larkin and Milne, 2017). In some cases, new health problems develop after caring ends, for example sleep and eating problems may develop and increased alcohol consumption is common. Interestingly though, some evidence suggests that carers of relatives with Alzheimer's disease may have higher levels of wellbeing than non-carers after the cared-for person's death. This may be linked to a 'sense of relief' and/or an increase in their 'sense of mastery' in terms of feeling confident about handling their life compared with managing all the challenges associated with their pre-bereaved state (Larkin and Milne, 2017).

The degree to which these legacies are experienced depends on a number of factors. More problematic caring experiences, such as those which involved a strained relationship with the cared-for person and very intensive caring, are linked to depression and lower levels of wellbeing (Larkin, 2009; Larkin and Milne, 2017). Recent work based on longitudinal studies about the role age plays (Tur-Sinai et al., 2022) shows that whilst middle aged carers' subjective ratings of health and financial capability improve, life satisfaction decreases. In contrast, ratings in all three areas decrease for older carers. This evidence underscores the complexity and nuanced individualised nature of both caring, and post-caring, life.

Support for former carers

The complex intersection of grief, loss and care-related legacies leave many former carers in a vulnerable position. Some need support to get back on their feet. Although former carers are beginning to have a more visible public profile, lack of policy recognition contributes to the very limited formal support that is available.

In addition to the (common) loss of social and informal support networks, former carers often have to contend with the withdrawal of support from statutory services. This routinely happens immediately post care home admission or the death of the cared-for person. This withdrawal can represent yet another loss – loss of (often) highly valued relationships with health or social care staff – exacerbating the carer's vulnerability (Cavaye and Watts, 2018). Once carers are no longer 'actively' caring, they are not regarded by local authorities as justifying 'assessments of need' or as being eligible for support. If a carer had joined a carers support group earlier in their care trajectory, they tend to continue to attend it post caring. Some third sector carers organisations offer specific groups to former carers and care homes may also provide support groups for relatives, such as a local Relatives and Residents Association. Although waiting lists can be an impediment, bereaved former carers may access bereavement counselling or support groups via organisations such as Cruse Bereavement Care (Milne and Larkin, 2023).

Several studies have addressed the fact that former carers have significant unmet needs and would benefit from a number of specific interventions (Cavaye and Watts, 2018). Key suggestions made to date include:

• the holistic assessment of practical and psychological needs for bereaved former carers. Recognition of the high levels of burden that carers supporting a relative with terminal conditions experience has prompted the development of comprehensive, holistic and person-centred assessments in national palliative and end-of-life services (Ewing and Grande, 2018). Such assessments could usefully inform local authority, voluntary sector and heathcare assessment of fomer carers' needs.

- the allocation of resources for formal targeted, proactive and needs-based post-caring support. This could include having a 'mentor' to support the transition from active caring to becoming a former carer (e.g., someone who has experienced this transition).
- specific groups for former carers run by third sector carers support agencies to cater for the specific challenges facing former carers, offer advice about practical issues (e.g., finances), and help them (re)engage with social activities, friends and interests.

Critical to the effectiveness of any extension of assessment and provision of support into carers' post-caring lives is recognition that the number of serial carers is increasing. Recent work by Keating et al. (2019) about caring across the life course highlights the nuanced connectivity between episodes of caring and potential cumulative outcomes. They underscore a need for carefully tailored support for those who transition in and out of caring over their life course.

Researching, conceptualising and theorising former carers' experiences of grief and loss

The evidence reviewed in this chapter clearly indicates that caring and post-caring experiences of grief and loss are interrelated. Some conceptual models of caring do incorporate a post-caring phase (Larkin and Milne, 2017). There are also a number of models which focus exclusively on the post-caring phase. In her work on bereaved carers, Larkin (2009) developed the concept of a post-caring trajectory comprising three phases. The first two are the 'post-caring void' and 'closing down the caring time', while the third, 'constructing life post-caring', involves getting life together again, during which former carers reconnect with their families, pursue their interests and take up new activities. Although Cronin et al. (2015) do not use the term 'trajectory' in their study of former carers whose relatives have either died, or been admitted to a hospice or care home, they conceptualise the post-caring period as a time of being 'between worlds', during which former carers experience three iterative interrelated transitions. These transitions have congruence with Larkin's (2009) model and are described as 'loss of the caring world', 'living in loss' and 'moving on'.

Useful as they are, existing models do not provide insights into the complexities of former carers' grief and loss and do not extend understanding about the support former carers may need to deal with these experiences. In part, this can be explained by the absence of conceptual granularity in models of caring, including post-caring frameworks. One way forward is to draw on conceptual models linked to grief, the best known being that of Kubler-Ross (1969), which identifies five common stages of grief – denial, anger, bargaining, depression and acceptance. Despite criticisms of this model, its incorporation into post-caring frameworks could both extend understanding of former carers and inform the development of support services.

Research about former carers also lacks analytical depth. A primary weakness relates to limited consensus about how a 'former carer' is defined. Although sub-populations of former carers have been identified, evidence about the different sub-groups is very uneven. Some groups of former carers are far less visible than others, in particular those who become former carers when the cared-for person goes into hospital, recovers from their health problem or goes into remission. Other groups are invisible, for example, those who do not fit the traditional model of family carer, such as ex-partners, and those who are former carers because they have chosen not to continue to care (Larkin and Milne, 2017).

Another challenge of existing research is its methodological limitations. That most studies are small-scale and conducted by different bodies (e.g., third sector organisations, independent think tanks) undermines the additive capacity of research. There is also minimal cross-fertilisation of ideas or expertise. Studies are (often): limited geographically; use small and unrepresentative sample groups and/or focus on one particular group of former carers (e.g., those who have cared for a relative with dementia); do not allow relationship differentiation with the cared-for person (e.g., caring relationships between spouses or between a parent and a son or daughter); and fail to identify 'serial' former carers. Opportunities to increase knowledge about the post-caring experiences of former carers are also constrained because there are few longitudinal studies. Most research takes a snapshot in time approach or captures post-caring experiences over a short period. Additionally, as former carers tend to be excluded from clinical studies of major co-morbidities (e.g., dementia and Parkinson's), a key opportunity to capture their experiences and perspectives is lost. Few funding sources are a limitation too. The evidence base is also fragmented and atomised (Kelleher and McGrath, 2016; Cavaye and Watts, 2018; Watts and Cavaye, 2018).

More fundamental deficits are linked to the absence of a theoretical lens of analysis. As post-caring tends to be conceptualised by 'adding' a 'former carer stage' to the end of the caring trajectory, a bifurcated model of carer/former carer is created (i.e., that a carer *actively provides care,* and a former carer is *no longer caring)*. This not only limits development of the conceptual status of former carer but also constructs 'formerality' as a single fixed state. Dementia caring illustrates the limitations imposed by this model well. Evidence suggests that dementia carers' journey from 'carer' to 'former carer' may involve at least two overlapping stages of formerality. When the person with dementia enters a care home, the carer's status becomes that of former carer. However, when the person with dementia dies the carer's status shifts into a 'new' type of former carer, that of bereaved former carer. This experience of status-shift involves a series of transitions, rather than a single transition from one status to another, as suggested by the bifurcatory model (Roland and Chappell, 2015). Other caring experiences also challenge this unidirectional model. For example, carers of relatives regularly admitted to hospital; a carer in this situation may move in and out of being a carer and former carer. Carers who support a spouse in the community and a parent in a care home do not fit either as they simultaneously occupy both statuses.

Knowledge about former carer experiences of grief and loss is limited and is constrained by conceptual, methodological and theoretical weaknesses. One way forward is to adapt theoretical and conceptual analyses from the wider carers field (e.g., life course analysis, the ethic of care, emotional labour, social liminality,

132   M. Larkin and A. Milne

biographical disruption and social identity) to add depth, breadth and granularity to our understanding of loss and grief amongst former carers.

Concluding comments

As demonstrated in this chapter, we do have some understanding of former carers' experiences of grief and loss in that there have been explorations of some significant issues. These include loss of the carer role once active caring ceases, finding a post-caring identity and role, some of the complexities of the grieving process for carers, and the intersection of caring and post caring experiences – the legacies of caring. However, this body of work is both narrow and conceptually confined and there is scope for substantial development. Further work identified focused around extending understanding of former carers' lives and roles by opening up discourse that is situated outside of the care trajectory. Central to this is discourse that can accommodate models of loss, grief, transition and identity drawn from other fields, and take account of the complexity of care, the life course, and the fact that carers may be exposed to losses associated with a caring role more than once. There is also a need to develop effective services and support for the distinctive needs of former carers. There is a related need to address theoretical and conceptual deficits and invest in new, and different types of, research in order to generate new knowledge, inform policy and service development and meet the specific and nuanced needs of former carers.

References

Carers UK (2019) *Facts about Carers*. London: Carers UK. Available at: www.carersuk.org/media/5w2h3hn2/facts-about-carers-2019.pdf (accessed 6 February 2024).

Carers UK (2021) *10 Facts about Loneliness and Caring in the UK for Loneliness Awareness Week*. London: Carers UK. Available at: www.carersuk.org/news/10-facts-about-loneliness-and-caring-in-the-uk-for-loneliness-awareness-week/ (accessed 6 February 2024).

Cavaye, J. & Watts, J.H. (2018) 'Former carers: Issues from the literature', *Families, Relationships and Societies*, 7, pp. 141–157. Available at: https://doi.org/10.1332/2046743 16X14676464160831.

Cronin, P. et al. (2015) 'Between worlds: The experiences and needs of former family carers', *Health and Social Care in the Community*, 23(1), pp. 88–96. Available at: https://doi.org/10.1111/hsc.12149.

Eloniemi-Sulkava, T. et al. (2002) 'Emotional reactions and life changes of caregivers of demented patients when home caregiving ends', *Aging and Mental Health*, 6(4), pp. 343–349. Available at: https://doi.org/10.1080/1360786021000006965.

Ewing, G. and Grande, G.E. (2018) *Providing Comprehensive, Person-Centred Assessment and Support for Family Carers Towards the End of Life: 10 Recommendations for Achieving Organisational Change*. London: Hospice UK. Available at: www.hospiceuk.org/docs/default-source/What-We-Offer/Care-Support-Programmes/Research/carers-report---10-recommendations-for-achieving-organisational-change_final.pdf?sfvrsn=0 (accessed 6 February 2024).

Geerlings, A.D. et al. (2022) 'Using former carers' expertise in peer support for carers of people with Parkinson's Disease', *NPJ Parkinsons Disease*, 8, 133. Available at: https://doi.org/10.1038/s41531-022-00381-0.

Greenwood, N. and Smith, R. (2019)) 'Motivations for being informal carers of people living with dementia: A systematic review of qualitative literature', *BMC Geriatrics,* 19(1), 169. Available at: https://doi.org/10.1186/s12877-019-1185-0.

Hughes, N., Locock, L. and Ziebland, S. (2013) 'Personal identity and the role of 'carer' among relatives and friends of people with multiple sclerosis', *Social Science and Medicine,* 96, pp. 78–85. Available at: https://doi.org/10.1016/j.socscimed.2013.07.023.

Isham, L., Bradbury-Jones, C. and Hewison, A. (2020) 'Female family carers' experiences of violent, abusive or harmful behaviour by the older person for whom they care: A case of epistemic injustice?', *Sociology of Health and Illness*, 42(1), pp. 80–94. Available at: https://doi.org/10.1111/1467-9566.12986.

Isham, L., Bradbury-Jones, C. and Hewison, A. (2021) ' "This is still all about love": Practitioners' perspectives of working with family carers affected by the harmful behaviour of the older person for whom they care', *British Journal of Social Work*, 51, pp. 3190–3208. Available at: https://doi.org/10.1093/bjsw/bcaa129.

Keating, N. et al. (2019) 'Life course trajectories of family care', *International Journal of Care and Caring*, 3(2), pp. 147–163. Available at: https://doi.org/10.1332/2397882 19X15473079319309.

Kelleher, C. and McGrath, H. (2016) 'What comes next? Family carers' experiences of role and identity transition on cessation of the caring role', *Advances in Consumer Research*, 44, pp. 508–509.

Kirby, E. et al. (2022) '(How) will it end? A qualitative analysis of free-text survey data on informal care endings', *International Journal of Care and Caring*, 6(4), pp. 604–620. Available at: https://doi.org/10.1332/239788221X16357694113165.

Kubler-Ross, E. (1969) *On Death and Dying.* London: Routledge.

Larkin, M. (2009) 'Life after caring: The post-caring experiences of former carers', *The British Journal of Social Work*, 39(6), pp. 1026–1042. Available at: https://doi.org/10.1093/bjsw/bcn030.

Larkin, M. and Milne, A. (2017) 'What do we know about older former carers? Key issues and themes', *Health and Social Care in the Community*, 25(4), pp. 1396–1403. Available at: https://doi.org/10.1111/hsc.12437.

Larkin, M. and Milne, A. (2021) 'Knowledge generation and former carers: Reflections and ways forward', *Families, Relationships and Societies,* 10(2), pp. 287–302. Available at: https://doi.org/10.1332/204674319X15761550214485.

Larkin, M., Henwood, M. and Milne, A. (2022) 'Older carers and carers of people with dementia: Improving and developing effective support', *Social Policy and Society,* 21(2), 242–256. Available at: https://doi.org/10.1017/S1474746420000615.

Lloyd, L. (2006) 'A caring profession? The ethics of care and social work with older people', *British Journal of Social Work*, 36(7), pp. 1171–1185. Available at: https://doi.org/10.1093/bjsw/bch400.

Milne, A. (2023) 'Older women and domestic abuse: Through a glass darkly', *The Journal of Adult Protection*, 25(3), pp. 143–155. Available at: https://doi.org/10.1108/JAP-10-2022-0022.

Milne, A. and Hatzidimitriadou, E. (2003) ' "Isn't he wonderful?": Exploring the contribution and conceptualization of older husbands as carers', *Ageing International*, 28(4), pp. 389–407. Available at: https://doi.org/10.1007/s12126-003-1011-y.

Milne, A. and Larkin, M. (2023) *Family Carers and Caring: What It's All About.* Bingley, UK: Emerald.

Molyneaux, V. et al. (2011) 'Reconsidering the term "carer": A critique of the universal adoption of the term "carer" ', *Ageing and Society*, 31(3), pp. 422–437. Available at: https://doi.org/10.1017/S0144686X10001066.

Rapaport, J. and Manthorpe, J. (2008) 'Family matters: Developments concerning the role of the nearest relative and social worker under mental health law in England and Wales', *British Journal of Social Work*, 38(6), pp. 1115–1131. Available at: https://doi.org/10.1093/bjsw/bcm025.

Robinson-Whelen, S. et al. (2001) 'Long-term caregiving: What happens when it ends?', *Journal of Abnormal Psychology,* 110*(4),* pp. 573–584. Available at: https://doi.org/10.1037/0021-843X.110.4.573.

Roland, K.P. and Chappell, N.L. (2015) 'A typology of care-giving across neurodegenerative diseases presenting with dementia', *Ageing and Society,* 35, pp. 1905–1927. Available at: https://doi.org/10.1017/S0144686X1400066X.

Seltzer, M.M. and Li, L.W. (2000) 'The dynamics of caregiving: Transitions during a three-year prospective study', *Gerontologist,* 40, pp. 165–178. Available at: https://doi.org/10.1093/geront/40.2.165.

Spencer, D. et al. (2019) 'Fear, defensive strategies and caring for cognitively impaired family members', *Journal of Gerontological Social Work,* 62(1), 67–85. Available at: https://doi.org/10.1080/01634372.2018.1505796.

Tur-Sinai, A. et al. (2022) 'Cessation of care for frail older adults: Physical, psychological and economic outcomes for family carers', *International Journal of Environmental Research and Public Health,* 19(6), 3570. Available at: https://doi.org/10.3390/ijerph19063570.

Watts, J.H. and Cavaye, J. (2018) 'Being a former carer: Impacts on health and well-being', *Illness, Crisis and Loss*, 26(4), pp. 330–345. Available at: https://doi.org/10.1177/1054137316679992.

Index

Note: Page numbers in *italics* indicate figures, and page numbers in **bold** indicate tables in the text

abuse 127
aftereffects of caring 113
Age UK 23, 79, 85
Alzheimer's disease 4, 5, 65, 66, 71, 79, 81, 84, 129; *see also* dementia/dementia care
ambiguous loss xii, xiii, 1–13; Boss' principles for developing or learning tolerance for xiii, 1–4, 8–13; impact 1, 4–7; multiplicity 3; polarisation 7–8; resilience to 1–2; structural impact 1
anticipatory grief 98, 127; anticipatory loss *vs.* 127; dementia care 66, 67, 80–1, 86–7, 89
Anticipatory Grief Scale 66
anticipatory loss xiii, 27, 28, 30–1, 37, 38, 126–7; anticipatory grief *vs.* 127; dementia carers 127
Asian caregivers 61
athletic identity xiv, 41, 43–4, 49; *see also* physical activity (PA)
Atkins, L. 48–9
Attig, T. 58
Australia: Carer Gateway 111; Carer Recognition Act 111; former carers (*see* Australian former carers); informal carers 110–11; loss in trajectories out of caring 110, 112–19
Australian former carers 113–19; financial stress 113; loss of sense of belonging 119; socially isolation 113
Australian National Carer Survey 113

Basile, M.J. 19
Behaviour Change Wheel 49
bereaved carers 90, 112, 124, 126–7, 130; *see also* bereavement

bereavement 56, 118; care endings and 110, 111, 112; children in the context of (*see* children); dementia 80, 83, 85; emotional consequences 126; former carers 126–30, 131
Biddle, S. 48
biographical disruption xii, 41; concept 27–8; trajectories of 33
biographical expectations 54–5
Blandin, K. 85
Bluebond-Langner, M. 37
Bons-Storm, M. 67, 75
Boss, Pauline xiii, 1–4, 8–13
Bowlby, J. 56
Brannelly, T. 65–6
Braun, V. 46
Brooks, D. L. 49
Bury, Michael 27, 28

CALMER 3
Cao, V. 48
care endings 110, 111–20; bereavement and 110, 112; cultural and relational expectations 114–15; as a failure 114; freedom 115; grief and 112; guilt 115; health problems 128–9; learning to live again after 118; loss 113; opportunities lost 116–18; socially isolation 113
care partners 79–90; ambiguous loss 81–2, 87–8, 89; anticipatory grief 80–1, 86–7, 89; anxieties 84; disenfranchised grief 83, 88–9; end-of-life decisions 84; existential crisis 84; financial impacts 84; interviews and findings 85–9; stress 84; testimonies 85
carer(s) xii; ambiguous loss (*see* ambiguous loss); bereaved 90, 112, 124, 126–7,

136   *Index*

130; growing number of 123; healthcare professionals and role of 16–26; mother as (*see* live-in carer); negative emotional experiences 41; physical activity and 42–9; poorer physical health 42; self-care 8–9, 98, 103; social networks 103; *see also* former carers
Carer Gateway service model 111
Carer Recognition Act 111
Carer Support Group 58
caring: aftereffects of 113; legacies of 127–9; research on 123; serial 124; *see also* carer(s)
Carlin, V. 83
Cavaye, J. 124
children 94–106; being prepared for death of an adult xiv, 94–102; being supported and cared after death of an adult xiv, 102–6; caring for aging relatives 61; grief experience 104–5; immediate bereavement period and 102; security and stability of 103; *see also* life-shortening conditions (LSCs)
Christianity/Christians 61, 67–76; denominations across the UK **67**
churches 59, 60, 65, 67–76
Cicchelli, L. 20
Clarke, V. 46
Clinical Frailty Scale 28–9
Communication Empowerment Framework 85
Confucian belief 61
constructing life post-caring 130
constructivist Grounded Theory Method (cGTM) 27, 29
co-researchers as participants 44–5
Corey, K. L. 118
courtesy stigma 28
COVID-19 pandemic xiii, 28, 55, 57, 88; end-of-life plans and 35–6, 38
critical situation 27–8
Cronin, P. 130
Cruse Bereavement Care 129

Dahlborg Lyckhage, E. 112
data collection and analysis 30, 45–6; *see also* research
Davidson, S. 12
Davies, D. J. 65
death *see* bereavement
death studies 66–7, 74
dementia/dementia care xiv, 65, 127; anticipatory grief 66, 67,

80–1, 86–7, 89; churches and 65, 67–76; disenfranchised grief (*see* disenfranchised grief); as a dreaded disease 67; former carers and 112; social death 127; theology and faith in xiv, 65–76; *see also* care partners of people with dementia
Dementia Friendly Churches 75
discovering hope 10, 12
disenfranchised grief xii, xiv, 7, 54, 56, 79, 83, 86, 88–9; as lonely experience 59
Doka, K. J. 58
domestic abuse 127
Dominguez, K.M. 59
dual identity 20
Dual Process of Grief Model 54, 62–3

Educating for Inclusive, Caring Communities (EICC) 67
Eifert, E. 49
Empowered Carers sessions 85
Empowered Conversations course 85
end-of-life experience 94–106
end-of-life planning 35–6, 37
Epps, F. 75
ethics 30
Evans, S. 81
exercise *see* physical activity (PA)
extended family 17

filial piety 61
financial stress 113
finding meaning 10, 12
five stages of grief model 24–5, 57
former carers 110, 123–32; aftereffects of caring for 113; description of 123–4; emotional responses 124; grief 126–7; health problems 128–9; legacies of caring 127–9; loss of caring role and identity 124–6; performative roles 125; post-caring activities 126; research about 123, 124, 130–2; support for 129–30; *see also* Australian former carers; care endings
Frankl, V. 62, 89
Friedrich, R. 67
funeral director 102

Garand, L. 66
General Practitioner (GP) 17
George, D. R. 66
Giddens, A. 27–8
Gill, D. L. 49

Index 137

Gitterman, A. 58–9
giving back 105
Goffman, I. 28
good death 37–8; COVID-19 and 38
Gottlieb, L. 57
grief 56–9; anticipatory (*see* anticipatory grief); Covid-19 pandemic and 57; death and 56; disenfranchised (*see* disenfranchised grief); Kübler-Ross' five stages model 24–5, 57; learning from 25–6; lost opportunities 116–18; non-death losses and 56–7, 59; psychodynamic perspective 79–80; as a subjective experience 104; *see also* loss(es)
Guàrdia-Olmos, J. 66
guilt 43, 47, 48; care endings 115

Haley, W. E. 23
Harris, D. L. 41, 56–7, 59
Hawthorn Friendship Scale 113
healthcare professionals xiii, 16–26; clinical decisions 20–2; communication 18–19; conflict between roles 18, 20; dual identity and dilemmas 19–20; experience impacting 24–6; family expectations 23–4; language 19; privileged knowledge 18–19; protective role 20–2
health problems 128–9
Herklots, Helena 23
Higgs, P. F. 55
Hudson, R. E. 67, 75

identity 19–20; athletic xiv, 41, 43–4, 49; dual 20; former carers and loss of 124–6; *see also* healthcare professionals
informal carers 15, 55–6, 62; in Australia 110–11; *see also* carer(s); former carers
isolation 70, 83, 84, 90, 127; as a barrier to physical activity 47; social 70, 71, 75, 110, 113, 128; spiritual 71

Judeo-Christian tradition of lament 76

Katz, N.T. 19
Keating, N. 130
Kessler, D. 57, 89
Kevern, P. 67
Kiper, D. 82, 83
Knight, C. 58–9
Kosloski, K. 41

Krist, A.H. 19
Kubler-Ross, E. 24–5, 57, 130

lament, Judeo-Christian tradition of 76
langmut 2
Larkin, M. 130
Laslett, P. 55
Laurencelle, L. 49
learning from grief and loss 25–6
legacies of caring 127–9
life-shortening conditions (LSCs) xiii, 27, 28–38; loss of an idealised good death 35–7; loss of certainty and ontological security 30–2; loss of future(s) 33–5; loss of idealised notions of babies and parenthood 31, 32–3; parallel planning for 28, 33–5, 37; prognosis of 31–2
lifestyle choices 46
life-threatening conditions 27
liminality 37, 41, 112
Lindahl, B. 112
Lindemann, E. 66
Lindsay, R.K. 42, 43, 48, 49
live-in carer 54–63; dealing with loss 59–62; loss and grief encountered 56–9; sense of purpose 60–1
loneliness 103
loss(es): ambiguous (*see* ambiguous loss); of an idealised good death 35–7; anticipatory (*see* anticipatory loss); of caring role 124–6; of certainty and ontological security 30–2; dealing with 59–62; of future(s) 33–5; of idealised notions of babies and parenthood 31, 32–3; learning from 25–6; non-death 56–7; trajectories out of caring 110, 112–19; transitory 57; *see also* grief
LSCs *see* life-shortening conditions

MacArtney, J.I. 37
Malan, D.H. 85
McCurry, M. K. 118
McLeod, D. 20
Meaning Reconstruction Theory 54, 62
Michie, S. 48–9
Montgomery, R. 41
Moon, P. J. 66
mother as a carer *see* live-in carer
Murdoch, I. 81

Nathanson, A. 2
National Health Service (NHS) 28, 41
Nazi concentration camps 62

138 *Index*

New York University Caregiver
Intervention (NYUCI) 85
non-death losses 56–7
normalising ambivalence 10, 12
nuclear family 17

object constancy 81–2
Office for National Statistics 55
ontological security 28, 30–2, 117
The Open University Human Research
Ethics Committee 30

PA *see* physical activity
parallel planning 28, 33–5, 37
parenthood, loss of idealised notions of
32–3
Penson, M. 41, 44–50
Pepin, R. 85
Pérez-González, A. 66
performative roles of former carers 125
physical activity (PA) xiii–xiv; barriers to
43, 47–8; Carers UK on 42; defined
42; lifestyle choices 46; Piggin on
42; psychosocial experience of 42;
research and findings 44–9; self and 47,
49; socioecological model of barriers
and facilitators to *43*; sport transition
research 43–4
Piggin, J. 42, 49
polarisation 7–8
Polenick, C.A. 62
Pope, E.M. 45
Post, S. G. 67
post-caring role 124, 126, 132
post-caring trajectory 128, 130
post-caring void 111, 118, 130

reconstructing identity 10
reflective practice group 86
reflexive thematic analysis 46
reflexivity 45
Reifsteck, E. J. 49
Relatives and Residents Association 129
research 123; former carer 124, 130–2;
life-shortening conditions (LSC) 29–38;
physical activity (PA) 44–9
resolution 8
revising attachments 10
reweaving process 59
Rogers, M. 2

Sabyani, H. 15, 18
Scott, S. 119

self-care 8–9, 98, 103
self-fulfilling prophecy 66
self-preservation 15
sense of purpose 60–1
serial caring 124
Shut, H. 62–3
social death 65–6, 127
social isolation 70, 71, 75, 110, 113, 128
The Solitary (Carlin) 83
spiritual isolation 71
sport transition research 43–4
Stroebe, M. 62–3
support for former carers 129–30
Swinton, J. 67, 72, 75

*The Talking, Telling, Sharing Framework:
End-of-life* 97
Taylor, J. 82
tempering mastery 12
Theological Education Institutes (TEI)
67–8
theology and dementia care xiv, 65–76;
death studies 66–7, 74; *see also*
Christianity/Christians
think out loud technique 45
trajectories out of caring 110, 112–19
Travellers to Unimaginable Lands
(Kiper) 82
triangle of conflict 85
Trudeau, F. 49

University of Aberdeen Committee for
Research Ethics and Governance in
Arts, Social Sciences and Business 68
unpaid care xii, 41, 138

van Gennep, A. 41
Vilajoana-Celaya, J. 66
virtues of caring 115
void 118; *see also* post-caring void

Walking the Tightrope (Age UK with
Carers UK) 23
Watts, J.H. 124
West, R. 48–9
Williams, S. 67
withdrawal of support 129
Woods, B. 67
World Health Organisation (WHO) 42, 48

Yao, P.L. 49
Young Women with Cancer Support
Group 58

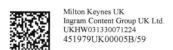
Milton Keynes UK
Ingram Content Group UK Ltd.
UKHW031330071224
451979UK00005B/59